Praise for *Walking Gone Wild*

Dami Roelse's love for the simple act of walking will inspire you to set out—for a stroll, a hike, or maybe even a hiking journey. Blending anecdote, trail musings, and step-by-step instructions, her book is a glorious and effective invitation to join her. She clearly has led many a non-walker out onto the trail, has recovered from missteps and has savored the delight of newly found vistas. If you have hiked in the past, you will remember why you loved it. If you have not been a walker or hiker, *Walking Gone Wild* may be your first irresistible invitation to saunter out.

Deborah Gordon, MD,
Northwest Memory Care, Madrona Health Care

Reading this book made me want to get the lead out, strap my boots on, and go walking and exploring. Dami's mix of philosophical musings, technical advice, personal insights into aging and loss and how to overcome their effect with mindful walking should encourage those looking for new inspirations to do the same.

Marielke Funke, Physical Therapist

Walking Gone Wild

How to Lose Your Age on the Trail

Walking Gone Wild

How to Lose Your Age on the Trail

Dami Roelse

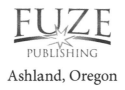

FUZE
PUBLISHING

Ashland, Oregon

Book design by Ray Rhamey, crrreative.com

Illustrations by Jack Wiens, jackwiens.com

ISBN 978-0-9998089-2-4

Library of Congress Control Number: 2018933634

Contents

To my father, who roused us kids on summer vacations before dawn to go "douwtrappen," walk in the dunes as the sun came up, and meet the new day with all its adventures.

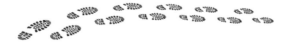

Acknowledgments

Writing *Walking Gone Wild* has taken stamina, humility, and a readiness to engage with the creative force—the same attributes demanded by the trail. Whenever I found myself stuck mid-draft, I remembered moments on the trail when I felt I would never reach a shady spot. I remembered scanning the terrifying Sierra Nevada mountains for the first time and thinking I could never hike way up there, then discovering that much is possible, one step at a time.

I wrote this book one step at a time, to share what I have learned in my walking life, and to encourage women to explore a new and surprising perspective on later life. I have shared my drafts in bits and pieces with my local writer friends, Jenni Egan, Kate Hannon, Stephanie Raffelock, Geri Hill, Janet Sola, and Alissa Lukara, a fabulous circle of knowledgeable and supportive writer women 50+.

Not only were they inspired to walk more, but they helped me tie my walking passion to a vision grander than just a brief handbook for the backpacking classes I was teaching locally. Thank you, dear sisters, for dreaming big with me.

Jack Wiens, the book's illustrator, helped me navigate the new territory of getting from words to pictures with patience, understanding, and grace. Thank you, Jack, for demonstrating how a picture is worth a thousand words.

Author, mentor, publisher, and local literary wiz, Molly Tinsley deserves credit for getting me to explore my writer self, first in classes, then in a focused writing group, and intermittently over tea. Thank you, Molly for taking on this book, introducing me to your publishing partner, Karetta Hubbard, and working away at changing my native Dutch grammar mistakes and making suggestions for more fluid expression. Thank you, Karetta, for introducing me to the gruesome process of reworking content to fit public scrutiny and interest. The process reminded me of packing my backpack for a long-haul trip, groaning at all the necessary stuff that can't possibly fit in! And then in the end, by trimming and reconsidering, it all fits, and the pack feels fine on my back.

I must also thank professional copy editor Laurel Robinson and my hawk-eyed book reviewers, Valeria Breiten, Leslie Black, Katy Bowen, and Deborah Gordon for cogent suggestions. I also want to thank Ray Rhamey for skillfully packaging *Walking Gone Wild*, helping me assess design choices I didn't know existed.

We live in the digital age. Even though I encourage a vacation from social media and the ever-present smartphone on the trail, I want to thank all the women who have expressed their enthusiasm and trepidations about walking and hiking through the online magazines I write for, *Sixty and Me* and

Trek magazine, and through my Facebook page, walkingwomen50plus. I owe a lot as well to the social media pages that allow hiking enthusiasts to communicate with one another across the world, such as the PCT Section Hikers; Women of the PCT; All Women All Trails—Hiking and Backpacking; and 52 Hikes in 52 Weeks.

Last but not least, I want to thank my children and their spouses, Yaro and Lena, Quinn and Michael, and Leela and Spencer for encouraging me in my solo hiking endeavors and for trusting me on the trail as long as I have my GPS device with me. I felt your trust continue as I ventured into my writing career, and it helps me focus on doing my job well. Thank you, dear ones, for believing in me! I hope you will keep a copy of *Walking Gone Wild* around for when you're of an age that you might need a reminder about living life deeply. I hope that your children, my grandchildren, will one day understand what drove their Oma to walk and hike.

Disclaimer

The information in this book is meant to supplement, not re-place, proper physical training when undertaking a walking, hiking or backpacking program. Like any activity involving balance and environmental factors, walking, hiking, and back-packing poses some inherent risk. The authors and publisher advise readers to take full responsibility for their health and safety and know their limits. Before engaging in activities de-scribed in this book, be sure that you are in proper physical condition, your equipment is well maintained, and you do not take risks beyond your level of experience, aptitude, training, and comfort level.

Preface

Do you look in the mirror, and wonder, "Where did *the real me* go?" Maybe you recall your twenty-year-old self in belted waistlines or sleeveless shirts. And skirts—remember them? Meanwhile, your current wardrobe features baggy pullovers, jeans or slacks, and jackets designed to hide your expanding backside. Perhaps your body looks the same, but you notice your energy is not the same as it was when you were younger. Thus you find yourself opting for the sofa instead of movement, the indoors instead of the outdoors, chomping chips instead of walking trips.

If any of these possibilities resonate for you, I invite you to join me on a trip, *Walking Gone Wild*. Supported by this guide, you will maintain and improve your physique, lift your spirits, and even make new friends.

Walking doesn't involve elaborate equipment or require large outlays of money. Yet it offers countless benefits to well-being: expanded physical and mental health and opportunities for adventure and accomplishment. So why do we avoid doing it? We can't find the time. The weather never seems to cooperate. We can't find the right shoes. The dishwasher didn't work this morning. There may be physical limitations that restrict walking or create discomfort, but there's a strong chance that you can work around them to develop a lifestyle that incorporates a healthy dose of movement into old age.

In my native Holland, walking and bicycling are regular daily activities. When I immigrated to the United States as a young woman, I was eager to embrace a new culture, its ease of living, and its opportunities for new experiences. But I noticed with bewilderment that Americans relied on their automobiles to go everywhere.

Whenever I could, I tried to continue my old habit of self-locomotion. I left my car parked and walked or biked to do my daily errands. I made an effort to explore nature's abundance in this vast country and discover its wild side in regular hikes and excursions. Now as I move into senior status, I can appreciate the tremendous positive effect these efforts have had on my life.

Even though I always engaged in some form of "sport" throughout my life, I had never considered walking an activity that could keep me healthy both mentally and physically, until life threw me a curveball with my husband's illness. Walking alone or with a close friend became my go-to way of processing the difficulties in my life. Because my neighborhood and town were and are conducive to walking, I went everywhere on foot.

When I lost my husband as a partner, I went for a long walk in the Himalayas, my spiritual home back when I was in my twenties. I needed to figure out what to do with my life. There I discovered the life-giving qualities of walking and hiking. Walking became my new "practice," a way of living mindfully, in balance. At the same time it enhanced my health and lowered my carbon footprint. Ten years later I've become a walking enthusiast and inspire those around me to add more walking to their lives.

This book tells not only my walking story but also the stories of women past 50 who have put walking into their lives. The stories are about real events and living people. I have changed names and circumstances to protect their privacy. Little-known facts gleaned from research will encourage you further to become a walking woman. Often dedicated walkers become avid hikers and then adventurous backpackers or long-distance hikers. Though there is no pressure to keep expanding your distances, the appendix includes training schedules for doing so carefully and safely.

Based on my decade of walking, hiking, and backpacking, I will hold your (reading) hand as you bring up your reservations and doubts about launching into this self-nurturing project. I hope to share your goals and successes. My goal is to motivate you to overcome whatever barriers hold you back and keep you indoors waiting to tackle the outdoors for whatever your reason. My Facebook page, WalkingWomen50plus, invites comments, including the good, the bad, and the ugly. Sharing your stories could motivate others to join us on the trails!

If you're inspired to walk more, to take up hiking or backpacking, this book can be your guide to doing so thoughtfully and safely. Remember, walking, hiking and backpacking are meant to add a positive dimension to your life, not become another chore you feel obligated to complete. My journey through our great outdoors has provided me with balance, a deep love for life, and inner peace.

Now is the right time to make the change and start, one step at a time. I encourage you to trust and enjoy *Walking Gone Wild*.

Ashland, Oregon, 2018

Section I

WALKING

What's a Woman to Do?

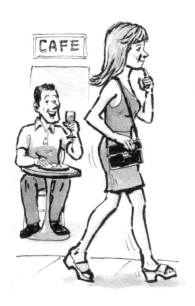

1: From Exercise to Mindfulness Practice

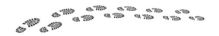

Walking brings health to mind and body. Walking allows for mindfulness

When I turned 65, I wanted to know, in depth, the place where I lived. No more running off to foreign places to find my happiness. I had traveled all over the world yet ignored the place I called home beyond what I saw from a car window and occasional forays on short trips. I decided to walk the length of Oregon.

I was relatively fit at the time, so I figured I could walk for 3 or 4 weeks carrying a backpack. I had been rowing competitively for 6 years; I was used to 3- and 4-day backpacking trips in the summer and could carry up to 35 pounds. I exercised an hour and a half each day, doing a mixture of aerobic training and strength training. I believed in working my body hard for periods of time. I had a sedentary job; I sat 10 hours a day behind a desk or in a classroom, 4 days a week. I figured that if I had a good, hard workout in the morning, I could rest on my laurels the rest of the day. I arrived at work with an endorphin high, which lasted most of the day.

I'd become aware, though, of research that concludes that exercising one hour a day does not significantly improve health. Being active throughout the day—walking and carrying, hauling and digging, pounding and dancing—is more conducive to increased fitness and staying healthy.

On my trips in the Himalayas, I had met women and men of different ages walking long distances from village to village, often carrying large loads of goods to market—even sewing machines—to sell their wares and offer their skills. Young and old, they moved at a slow, but steady pace. They helped each other balance their loads, held on their backs with a strap that wrapped around their foreheads.

In India I met women carrying stones and bags of sand on their heads, from the beach to a building site. They walked gracefully, holding their necks straight. From these travels, I gathered that walking with a load doesn't have to be torture if you balance the load on your body. I also saw that walking can be a community-building affair that brings people together. People talked, shared news, and shared their homes with travelers from other regions.

I was setting out on a journey to test these facts of health and community building, to experience how walking day in, day out with a load would change my body. I learned that, as with Asian villagers, walking the American wilderness brings people together as a community. Hikers stop and share information about the trail, the river crossings, the snowpack.

They help each other stay safe and share their delight in the surrounding beauty. I learned that walking and carrying a balanced load with all my belongings gives a degree of freedom, autonomy, and confidence I had never experienced.

I also experienced the effect of walking on my mind. In the Himalayas, I had met locals with prayer wheels, walking and praying as a way to prepare for a good afterlife. Now I know that the rhythm of walking is conducive to meditation and brain health.

One study of a group of middle-aged adults had them take three 40-minute walks a week for a year. At the end of the period, MRI scans verified that the hippocampus in their brains—a part of the limbic system, associated with memory, emotions, and motivation—had grown on average by 2 percent. The hippocampus gets smaller when we hit our mid-50s, which leads to an increase in memory loss.

Just as meditation increases the mind's ability to focus, walking focuses the brain. When I hiked at high altitude and in difficult terrain, this increased concentration became even clearer. In the thin air, all I could do was breathe and pay attention to moving my feet one step at a time. I suspect that the single-minded focus mustered by high mountain climbers to reach their goal is a good part of what attracts them to climbing.

In the documentary film *Meru*, the interviewer asks climber Conrad Anker why he keeps going back to the mountains, having lost his best friend and climbing partner to them, and knowing he could lose his own life. Anker answers by citing the heightened focus of climbing, which creates a feeling of expansiveness and connectedness in the brain few pleasures can rival, a "mountain high."

I'm not suggesting that high-mountain climbing is the only way to experience this complex feeling. Sitting in meditation you can reach the same place. But why not get the double advantage of an expansive mind and a healthy body by taking up walking and hiking? As Sayadaw U. Silananda points out in his article, "The Benefits of Walking Meditation," "Walking meditation can help us gain insight into the nature of things, and we should practice it as diligently as we practice sitting meditation or any other form of meditation."

Health, community, confidence, and meditative connection can be achieved by taking up walking. Let's see how, in more detail, in the chapters that follow.

2: Women by the Water

Sweat pouring off our faces, we unsnapped our backpacks, let them slide onto the ground, and, freed from the weight, sat down against the flaking red bark of a madrone tree (*arbutus menzieisii*), our eyes on the beauty before us. A grove of trees surrounded us, birds chirped in the limbs above us, and ten feet away, water rushed between the stones in the small creek. After sitting there for a few minutes, we looked at each other and nodded.

With energy we couldn't believe we still possessed, we pulled ourselves back up and headed for the creek. Settling on rock outcroppings, we untied our shoes, peeled off our dusty socks, and let our tired, sore feet delight in the chill of rushing water. "Ah, we made it!"

It was at least 98 degrees Fahrenheit that afternoon. As our heels cooled in the icy stream, so did our bodies. By the time we'd finished the last of our trail mix, our bodies could enjoy the warmth of the rocks underneath us.

Nearby, a group of women were watching their children splash and jump. Apart from the group, perched on a granite boulder watching us, was a woman who looked to be in her early forties. She was dressed in loose clothing, an oddity among the others in shorts and tank tops. We nodded her way, but, still giddy with accomplishment, continued chatting about our 4-day adventure, the heat while we climbed to 6000 feet, the thunderstorm in the night, the cold bath at Sheep Springs, the silent green canopy as we made the long descent into the Ashland watershed leading us to this spot at the far end of Lithia Park. Absorbed in our conversation, we didn't notice her get up and move toward us.

"May I ask you a question?" her soft voice inquired.

I turned toward her. "Sure."

"Are you thru-hikers?" She was referring to those hiking long stretches or the entire Pacific Crest Trail (PCT). Many chose our friendly town as a spot to stop and refuel.

"Not yet," I told her. "We just walked four days from Cook and Green Pass, in California, back to Ashland where we live. We're training for a longer hike we want to do later this summer."

"You two look so happy and strong."

"We are happy," I said. "Hard not to be when we can still get around like this at our age."

Tears welled and ran down her cheeks. "I am envious of your aliveness, your vigor. I feel like my body is deserting me. No energy. My children are almost teenagers." She pointed toward the group of older kids playing down the creek a way. "Is it possible to be over the hill at 40?"

"You think *you* are over the hill?" my friend said to her. "No, no, we just came over that hill." My friend pointed at Mount

Ashland and grinned. "We are the ones who are over the hill. We're in our sixties."

"What is your magic bullet? Is there a pill I can swallow? I want to be happy with myself again."

"No magic bullet, no pill," I said. "Just walking. Why not give it a shot? It might give you back your confidence. When you feel good, you don't have time to worry about your age. See how sweaty and dirty we are? We don't care." Thus I offered my simple walking remedy, the remedy I'd shared with many other women, women I was now taking onto the trail, training them to become confident long-distance hikers.

The woman smiled at us now, "Okay, you two inspire me."

"We're glad," I said, smiling back. "If you stay active, I predict many good years ahead for you."

We put our grubby socks and hiking shoes back on and hoisted the not-so-heavy packs to walk the last mile home to a shower and a clean bed for the night. Smiling now, the woman waved, and then strolled over to a group of women that opened to include her.

I wished I could have handed her my business card to connect her with a backpacking course I offer. But I don't carry them with me when I'm hiking—it adds too much weight. I wanted more time to emphasize to her that her confidence would return, along with a sense of wholeness just at that time in her life when she thought she was losing it.

The Pacific Crest National Scenic Trail is a wilderness footpath and equestrian route designated in 1968 under the National Trail Systems Act. The trail runs from Mexico to Canada along a crest of the Sierra Nevada mountains in California and the Southern and Northern Cascades in Oregon and

Washington state. My hiking companion and I had just covered one small segment of its length. When we reached our destination—the Cascade-Siskiyou trailhead leading to Ashland—we gave each other big high fives, and the glow of completion and endorphins mixed into big, sunscreen-streaked grins on our faces. If ever cars disappeared from the planet, we knew we could haul our belongings and walk to where we wanted to go. Creating a graduated golden hue in the sky, the sun began its descent for the day. The air was pure and fresh with early summer. We knew our journey would never be over. The trail had stolen our hearts.

3: The Magic of 50

The disheartened woman by the creek was experiencing a natural development as her mothering and childbearing years were ending. She no longer saw herself as an attractive female and much-needed nurturer. Thanks to improvements in living conditions and health care however, a woman's life doesn't end when she's past her childbearing years. As psychologist Linda Savage notes in "The Three Stages of a Woman's Life," "The ancient tripartite divisions of Maiden, Mother, and Crone can be even more meaningful in women's lives as the Crone stage becomes one third of our lifespan." It requires a change in consciousness to experience this part of our life in its full richness.

This change in outlook does not evolve automatically or easily as demonstrated by the initial chagrin of my friend Kathy:

"Fifty Is Nifty!" shouted the banner hanging from the ceiling at the entrance to her dining room. But Kathy sat in the Barcalounger in the living room with her hands blocking her view of the cheery sign. She was wondering, *How did I get here so quickly? Just the other day I was running after two kids, making lunches before breakfast, kissing their little faces as they waited for the school bus, then heading off to the office.* Life had seemed without end. Fifty sounded old and scary. She wondered where her happy face would come from when her friends began arriving to help her celebrate the big 5-0. How would she shake the blahs?

As her friends paraded into the house with their favorite foods personally prepared for the half-century celebration, all she could think was *What do I do next? My best me is in the rearview mirror. My future is lost to my past.* Her pity party was replacing her birthday party.

After the candles were blown out and the cake was consumed, the ritual smart-aleck remarks began. One by one, they promoted the unfavorable side effects of old age:

You know you are getting old when it takes you two tries to get up from the couch.

You know you are getting old when you actually want socks for Christmas.

You know you're old when "getting a little action" means your prune juice is working!

I'd rather be over the hill than under it.

You know, you know, you know. The evening couldn't end quickly enough.

The next day I went over with an exotic Japanese powdered tea and teacups. "I couldn't help but notice you weren't having a good time last night," I said.

"Well, I admit I was freaking out," Kathy said. "I feel as though the clock just started ticking at a faster rate. I grab the moment, but I can't seem to hold on to it. Time used to be my friend helping me decide what comes next. But now it seems nothing comes next."

"Age is not important unless it is cheese," I said. "Someone famous said that, but don't ask me to remember who."

Kathy finally smiled.

"Sorry I'm being such a downer," she said. "I really can't complain. I'm healthy. I have a job I like."

"Yeah, the change can put you in a mood," I admitted. "You may want to take ahold of that with some exercise." I knew how important it had been for me to exercise to stabilize my mood during menopause. Kathy listened to what I said, and it didn't take long before she made changes. One resolution she made was to take up walking.

This book is for you if, like Kathy, you want to explore new ways of living after 50 and foster the experience of a long, fulfilling life.

As the hormones change in our bodies around menopause, feelings about ourselves fluctuate. Menopause can cause weight gain, sleep troubles, and mood swings, setting the stage for negative thoughts about our appearance. Measuring ourselves against images of other, good-looking and younger women may reinforce these negative thoughts and feelings. If we concentrate on moving our bodies, that kind of body awareness can reshape how we feel about ourselves. Subtle emotional changes will occur, and as we continue being active, we have more control over our thoughts. We can focus on identifying personal objectives and achieve them.

Here's the good news! After menopause, as hormones stabilize, negative feelings abate and self-content becomes the norm. In the article "Menopause and Mood Disorders," Stacey Gramann notes that "studies of mood changes during menopause have generally revealed an increased risk of depression. But there can be a decrease in risk during postmenopausal years."

As women past 50 we can experience a greater sense of well-being and a renewed feeling of energy. We are freed from the distraction of biology and the imperative to find a mate and procreate. In fact, in Native American tradition, a woman is not fully grown until she reaches the age of 52!

The manner in which we live our lives, especially the last third of our lives, affects everything, including the way we pass on. Psychologist Linda Savage puts it this way:

> It is not that we are completely done with the past or with the roles that we played, but we are now able to turn our life experience (both the wounds and the triumphs) into wisdom. We are ready to make our contribution, our special calling. This is the path of power. This is the true purpose of the Wise Woman Stage.

Thus we can choose to have creation still take place after menopause; it simply takes a non-biological form. The time is finally available to paint, teach, start a new business, spend time with grandchildren, and yes, walk, hike and backpack. Women can focus on what they really want to experience, learn, and contribute to the world. In other words, at this age, a woman's life offers the opportunity for healing and completion through creativity and healthy activity. As Sara Lawrence-Lightfoot observes in *The Third Chapter, Passion, Risk and Adventure in the 25 Years After 50,* "We must develop a compelling vision of later life: one that does not assume a trajectory of decline after fifty, but one that recognizes it as a time of change, growth, and new learning; a time when 'our courage gives us hope."

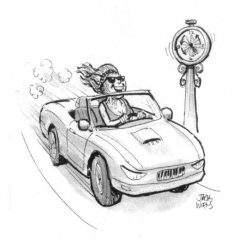

Putting Aging into Reverse

We can't change the fact that we age. If we're lucky, we have a partner who will age with us, appreciate the depths of our inner being,
and find us lovable. Many men, however, succumb to the biologi-
cal drive of chasing an attractive, younger woman. This leaves
women feeling depressed as they age or, at least, pressured to keep
a youthful physique. They turn to both external means and internal drive to conceal the aging process. Face-lifts, hair coloring,
body alterations, extreme diets, and harsh exercise routines are
presented to women as weapons in the battle against aging.

What's a woman to do when she isn't lucky enough to have
the means to keep herself looking young? Or perhaps she just
doesn't want to be pressured into appearing as something she
no longer is? She wants to be valued for her self, not her sex.

Many women try to keep up . . . until they give up. Until the
menopausal weight gain sticks its tongue out at them, and food
and wine are the immediate reward for feeling depressed. Until

their joints ache and watching a show on TV beats imitating men and women in shorts and leotards sweating away in an ultra-power-strength-building class at the gym.

To illustrate how real this dynamic is, let me offer a story from my own experience. I'd lost my husband at 59, and my children were grown and moving on in their lives. I missed having a partner for intimacy and companionship. I joined an online dating site. Although I was exercising, eating well, and looking 10 years younger than my age, as everyone was telling me, I still wasn't finding a man in my age category interested in exploring a relationship. I found only older males who, it seemed, needed a nurse, cook, or attentive company for their various stages of decline.

When I finally met a single man my age, through the dating site, I asked him how the response to his profile had been.

"Oh," he said, "every time I'm active online, I get 90 hits and have choices galore."

"Are these women your age?" I asked.

"All ages, many of them younger, but older ones also. My other single male friends have the same experience. There must be way more single women than men."

"Or more men choose younger women, limiting the pool of available age-compatible men," I said.

"You're right. Men date down in age," he said.

"I wonder how compatible a couple is when they differ 20 years in age, though," I said.

My new friend acknowledged that a much younger woman meant that compatibility could be questionable. The man and woman would be in different phases of life. To share lives, the (older) man might have to step back into a world of family, raising children, and providing. If a man was healthy, he could do so. But what about an older, graying woman at the end of her career matched with a younger male?

When I asked my friend how he maintained his physical prowess, he said, "I don't try very hard. When I look in the mirror, I see it—my skin, my body parts, it's all going south. But women don't seem to mind."

"Lucky you!" I said. "When an older woman looks in the mirror, she pulls and tugs at herself, then finally pulls out some torturous body harness and wiggles herself in so she can show off her curves through her clothes. If she doesn't do that, she is giving herself the verdict."

"The verdict?" My friend raised his eyebrows.

"Yes, the verdict says she is no longer attractive in the relationship market. The verdict says she is no longer valuable." I sighed and thought about all the woman struggling with relationships and self-image.

As we grow older, we lose partners, we struggle with our loneliness, we think we'll never be important to someone again. We hope that a man or woman will find us and make us happy. After my experience seeking a partner at an older age, however, I began to wonder whether a partner really is so crucial to happiness and well-being in the third stage. Maybe that search is a reflex, carried over from younger years. Maybe this later stage brings up the awareness that we are each responsible for our own happiness, partnered or not.

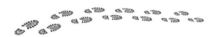

We must develop a compelling vision of later life: one that does not assume a trajectory of decline after fifty.

Making a Choice

If we feel the world doesn't appreciate us as women in the third phase of life, we may think we have only two choices: either reverse aging by working hard on our fitness and looks, or accept our loss of value and comfort ourselves by sliding onto the couch in front of the TV.

If we choose the couch, comfort foods, and entertainment, we are setting ourselves up to become an accelerated aging machine. We'll be embracing a habit that will erode not only our health but also our feelings of self-worth. If, on the other hand, we choose the skinny fitness classes, the Botox treatments, and the no-carbs-super-antioxidant-green-smoothie diet, we may become friends with stress and the creepy feeling of not being ourselves.

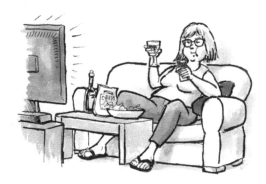

Either we will forget ourselves in the world of glorious stories on the screen while we're dipping into the ice-cream bucket to raise our dopamine levels, or we will learn to boost our self-esteem with envious comments from peers who don't have our stress-inducing self-discipline. As we dip in the ice-cream bucket, we will lose our ability to move comfortably because of the extra weight we've gained, and if we take extreme measures to keep the appearance of age at bay, we may lose our happy, carefree laugh because of the constant, gnawing stress.

I know I'm painting a radical, worst-case picture, but if some of these suggestions echo your thoughts even a little, there is a way out of the morass of diminishing self-esteem. There are other ways to feel good and alive. One of them is adopting a walking life. The walking life is more than taking a walk every day. The walking life means embracing ourselves, putting ourselves first, and giving ourselves the happiness we deserve.

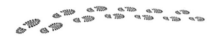

A walking life means embracing yourself—putting yourself first.

4: Why Walk?

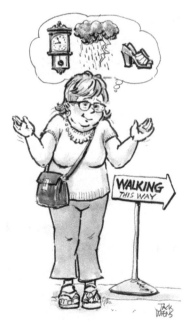

Women learn how to sit. Sit in school, sit in offices, sit in cars as they commute, sit at home. And as Annie Dillard notes in *The Writing Life*, "How we spend our days is, of course, how we spend our lives." How do you spend your days? Do you feel good about it?

Excessive sitting affects our body's metabolic system. As Dr. James Levine of the Mayo Clinic observes in his book Get UP!, "Today, our bodies are breaking down from obesity, high blood pressure, diabetes, cancer, depression, and the cascade of health ills and everyday malaise that come from what scientists have named sitting disease."

People who work a sedentary job sit on average 10 hours a day, and it can be as high as 15 hours. The total counts commuting, sitting down for meals, and sitting down for some TV or game time for relaxation after work. An hour of exercise a day does not cancel out the harmful effects of this amount of sitting. You can calculate your sitting time online at Juststand. org, where you'll find the infographic "Sitting Disease."

Here's how too much sitting played out for a colleague of mine.

Even though she lived in a house in the country with a swimming pool and garden plot, Ellen didn't spend much time in the outdoors. As her children grew up, she drove them back and forth to school since the school bus didn't come out where they were.

As a working mom, she commuted 40 minutes to her job, where she sat behind her desk, saw clients, and supervised other clinicians. She'd get up to walk to the file room once in a while, or to bring a client in from the waiting room.

As she got older and the kids left the house, she would leave earlier in the morning after watching the dawn over a cup of tea. She'd hurry to avoid the traffic jam at the off-ramp in the town where she worked. In the evening after picking up some groceries, and making dinner, she was tired and sank into her comfortable chair to chat with her husband, read, or watch TV. The weekends were filled with social calls, work around the house, and at times seeing clients in her private practice. The garden turned into the never-ending chore of keeping weeds at bay instead of the pleasure of raising healthful food.

There was no time for formal exercise. She was a petite woman with little room for physical expansion. After menopause she gradually gained weight, a pound a year. Eating salads for lunch didn't help. She felt more and more tired and less energetic, and was thus less enthusiastic about attempting a physical workout. At 58, when she went in for her yearly physical exam, the doctor told her: "You have type 2 diabetes. You have to lose weight. Start exercising or you'll be on medication from now on."

Ellen had seen enough clients in her practice who were overweight, depressed, and unmotivated, and she knew she had to take her doctor's words seriously. Since she didn't want to add another trip into town to a gym, she decided to walk: every Saturday morning she walked the country road from her home toward town.

Farther and farther she walked. Once she had the Saturday habit of walking, she set a bigger goal to walk a marathon. She found ways to walk during her workdays and got up earlier to get some walking in; she walked during her lunch hour and trained for the big day. A year later she walked the marathon, while her family cheered her on. She didn't stop there. She kept walking, lost the necessary weight, and got her diabetes under control.

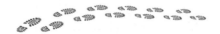

Walking is a return to a natural form of movement.

Of course not all physical problems can be solved with walking. There are a host of reasons, however—some more obvious than others—to choose walking and not some other activity to deal with the problems of aging and deteriorating health. The primary reason is that walking is a return to a natural form of movement. Walking is in our genes and good for our DNA. DNA is what holds the gene pattern underlying all our functions.

DNA molecules need to be stimulated regularly—renewed, you might call it—to express themselves and keep our bodily functions doing their job. Natural movement stimulates the DNA to "instruct" cells to build more cells that enable the body to function.

Like every animal moving about its territory, humans are meant to move about. Our bodies are designed to walk to gather our food, to hunt, and to find fertile living areas, and while doing so, to renew the DNA patterns embedded in our cells. It is a beautiful reciprocal relationship between cells.

In other words, our bodies are built to walk for survival. Not to swim or fly, not to sit staring at a computer screen or drive a car. When we walk, all our organs are stimulated, the load on our cells shifts, and the muscles start drawing nutrients necessary for good health into their cells.

Even though health professionals tell us to exercise an hour 3 times a week or walk 30 minutes a day, you can't fit all your need for cellular movement in even a 1-hour exercise session a day. You can't undo the damage of sitting most of the day with that same 1-hour session. Katy Bowman notes this in *Move Your DNA*:

> Motions that used to be incidental to living (recurring all day long) and cellular loads that used to be built into everyday life have been doled out—to computers, machines, and other people moving on our behalf. There is no way to recover the specific bends and torques, no way to recreate one hundred weekly hours of cell-squashing in seven, and no technology, at this time, smart enough to override nature.

We may not be able to create the life of constant movement Katy Bowman harkens back to, but we can add movement into our day by getting up more, walking more, shifting sitting locations (on the floor, on cushions and meditation benches), and standing or using a treadmill while computing .

Joy Through Walking

Yes, joy! Walking as a natural form of movement creates feelings of joy and contentment. It produces chemicals in the brain that foster a mild euphoria by flooding the brain with beta-endorphins, a self-made morphine-like chemical. Of course, there are passive ways of releasing such chemicals in the brain. Eating certain foods stimulates the release of pleasurable chemicals, although the relationship between certain foods and the release of certain neurotransmitters isn't fully known. However, ingesting food as a source of pleasure has its negative side effects, as the scale and your heavy breathing will tell you.

Mihaly Csikszentmihalyi, called Mihaly for short, is the architect of the concept of "flow," the creative moment when a person is completely involved in an activity for its own sake. Walking can be a vehicle to the state of flow, for when we walk, the stimulated brain will get new, creative ideas.

The creative state, the state of flow, gives meaning to our life. Mihaly found in his research that people who had the basics of living covered did not experience more or less happiness by acquiring more things.

Their happiness, instead, was tied to a state of ecstasy, a word derived from the Greek *ex-stasis,* meaning "standing next to or outside of." Ecstasy is not an all-out ecstatic, over-the-top happy state. It's an altered state, a state of being freed from ourselves, in which the body doesn't impede our experience of connectedness.

When people pursuing different activities describe the state of flow, they mention the total absorption in what they are doing, the sense of suspension of time and bodily needs for an uninterrupted period of time. It often happens spontaneously when we're doing something we love that deeply engages us. In that state of full engagement, we make discoveries and new connections, and we perform at our highest skill level. Einstein made his discoveries in a state of flow, a composer creates new music in a state of flow, I just hand-rolled the perfect tortilla in a state of flow! The experience of flow leaves a lasting euphoric feeling.

The more we experience flow, the easier it is to enter that state. The enhanced focus on our environment when we walk, the sense of rhythm that sets in when we walk a distance, the enhanced focus on breath and body when we climb at high elevation, all lead to a state of flow. Walking with awareness will get you to the creative state of flow.

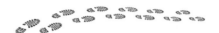

Walking with awareness will get you to the creative state of "flow."

Balancing the Body Through Walking

Walking doesn't have to be hard walking to have wonderful effects. It can be easy walking, and the amazing results of cell squashing will still be there. Focused exercise routines tend to work certain muscle groups repetitively, often overworking them in relation to other body parts. Such routines can become harmful to the body. Balanced walking, on the other hand, creates a movement wave in the spine, a wave that loosens every body part.

This discovery by Moshe Feldenkrais in the 1970s formed the basis of the Feldenkrais method of movement therapy. Feldenkrais exercises help people regain "original" movement by teaching in slow motion how to walk, or to sit down and get up again using muscles as they were designed to be used. Additionally walking aligns breathing with movement, providing the flow of oxygen to all the cells, creating a sense of well-being. These physical effects of walking are another reason to adopt this easy routine and make it a part of your life so that life becomes an experience of harmonious balance instead of a struggle with pain.

Reducing Stress Through Walking

Walking balances the body, and it reduces stress for body and mind. Other forms of exercise can do that also, you say, like yoga and water aerobics. But other forms of exercise have drawbacks. Yoga and water aerobics are not always available the way walking is, and they are not weight bearing. Other more aerobic, weight-bearing forms of exercise, such as kickboxing and CrossFit routines, can be performed for only short periods of time; if we attempted several sessions in a day, we might injure ourselves or be too fatigued to do anything else between sessions.

By contrast, we can walk for longer periods and multiple times a day with light rest periods in between without ill effect. Walking allows us to think and observe at the same time as the mind relaxes in a mildly euphoric state.

Exercise routines like kickboxing may create impressive strength results but not necessarily balance of body and mind. The bursts of chemicals released in intense exercise are addictive, leading us to crave more. Furthermore, extreme muscle development does not leave the body flexible, because it binds the muscles with its weight and contracted tissue and often invites injury or pain in later life. Lisa's story is an example of how super-fitness can create problems.

I shared an office with Lisa for several years, and because she had always been shy and I was much older, she opened up to me slowly. Our shared love for the outdoors was a conversation starter. Lisa told me she had hiked regularly as a teenager and that in college she had started running long distances to offset the hours of studying.

She sighed wistfully when she had to admit that with a job, a husband, and a young child, her time was too limited to go on long runs anymore. At the end of the workday several times a week, she would dash out to make it to a CrossFit class at the gym. I commented on her apparent muscle strength. "I wasn't always this way" she told me. "I used to be lanky and lean when I was running, but doing CrossFit has really built up my muscles."

Then changes at work and a child with frequent colds and poor sleeping patterns took their toll, and Lisa started complaining of stiffness, pain, and headaches. She missed work to deal with a sick child and felt even more stressed about her work performance. The strong muscles of her arms, neck, and back began to spasm and cause her a lot of pain.

Visits to the chiropractor didn't relieve the pain or the headaches she was experiencing. She would show up for work tired from lack of sleep. She developed allergies. Lisa demonstrated the dangers of pure strength development movement when it goes awry.

Developing strength and muscle is fine when it's done in a context of healthy, balanced movement, involving all parts of the body. But just bulking up without a balanced outlet for the strength makes for a tight body that cannot deal with stress very well and breaks down. Lisa had a road ahead of her to undo the damage and develop a more balanced, relaxing exercise routine. Walking became the go-to activity, for its combination of balanced movement and strength building.

Nonphysical Benefits of Walking

It's long been known that walking has social and creative benefits. A century ago Robert Walser's novella *The Walk (Der Spaziergang)* tells of a writer who describes what he encounters on a walk on an ordinary day in a small town. As the writer's ambling connects him with the world around him, it lifts him out of his solitary life. In a conversation with the local tax collector who wonders how he, the writer-walker can make a sufficient living, the writer-walker replies:

> "Walk, . . . I definitely must, to invigorate myself and to maintain contact with the living world, without perceiving which I could not write the half of one more single world, or produce the tiniest poem in verse or prose . . . Walking is for me not only healthy and lovely, it is also of service and useful . . . and spurs me on to further creation."

If we choose to walk alone instead of connecting with a person, we will connect with the world around us. Our environment will stimulate our thinking.

We can also walk while accomplishing tasks, such as carrying groceries, delivering garden bounty to a friend, or studying nature, collecting plants or mushrooms.

When we walk in the company of others, we enrich our social life. Inviting a friend for a walk is a gift of both a social visit and health. The social connections available through walking are particularly relevant for women of a certain age. In the United States and the developed world, women live longer than men and often spend their later years living alone. Whether we walk to avoid isolation and stay connected with our community, or to experience a connection with nature, we will find in walking an emotional lifesaver.

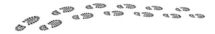

A walking life means pursuing many paths.

- Walk when you can.
- Move about more in your home or place of work.

- Use walking as a means of creating a state of flow.
- Walk as a way to create social connection.
- Walking and use movement as your first go-to to think.
- Walk to break up the sitting tasks of your day.
- Walk to wind down at day's end.

5: Adopting a Walking Mindset

I have always been passionate about living well. As I get older, I don't feel any less passionate. Maya Angelou's words have inspired me: "My mission in life is not merely to survive, but to thrive; and to do so with some passion, some compassion, some humor, and some style."

I didn't walk for health reasons, but I found health as I walked. I walked as an ecofriendly way of living, a habit left over from an almost carless childhood in a country where abundant, cheap public transportation kept the automobile from becoming an essential. As I grew up, I walked to school. I still remember the street leading up to my elementary school lined with mature chestnut trees, a green tunnel that dropped shiny brown chestnuts in fall. I walked to the train station, the bus, and the trolley stop, meeting and greeting people in my neighborhood on the way. I walked from the station to work, and to the university. I walked to the store to buy groceries and even had a shopping mall within walking distance. I didn't own a car until I moved to the United States in my mid-twenties and chose a rural home 5 miles from the nearest town.

Thus for the first third of my life, I managed without owning a car or using one on any regular basis. I count myself lucky to have had that experience, because I knew the pleasure of walking, meeting my community on foot, and having time to think about the issues of the day at school or work. I forced this experience to some extent on my children. I walked them 2 miles to school; I refused to drive them. I provided them with bicycles. They grumbled until they grew up and realized the benefits of the walking habit.

The power of my early life routine has influenced my adult life. Dr. Michael McCullough calls routines "mental butlers":

> Once you have a routine, the mental processes that stimulate the behavior take place automatically. You save time and energy and reduce stress by skipping the mental to-ing and fro-ing of making a decision, and slide directly into getting the task done. Instead of having to organize each day from scratch, routines create a framework for small decisions, and leave you with more time to devote to bigger decisions you have to make.

Americans who have grown up with cars drive them ev

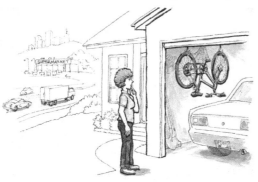

erywhere—to the store, to school, to work—and live where distances are great and transportation options few. They cannot imagine life without a car or using their bodies for transportation. Thus walking doesn't have the power of habit, at least not at first, and the choice gets overlooked and forgotten when time is short, the weather is unfavorable, the distance is more than a mile, or the roads lack safe sidewalks. It takes awareness and persistence to change a habit and develop a new routine. We must help each other do so.

When I walked to the gym for my weekly rowing workout during the winter, my rowing buddies greeted me with, "Good for you! You're already warmed up!"

When we finished up and headed out for coffee after the hour-long workout, I turned to walk to the cafe less than a mile away. Several people offered me a ride. I declined, telling them I liked to walk and cool down. Soon one woman joined me in my walk and left her car parked at the gym.

Within a few weeks several women were walking to coffee and back to their cars. They had broken the habit of getting into their cars for every short distance. I now routinely invite friends to walk to the theater together for a show, or to walk the extra miles to a meeting point, and my walking habit is catching on with others around me.

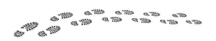

It takes awareness and persistence to change a habit and develop a new routine of walking.

Making the Change

Are you motivated to walk more? You don't have to swear off sitting altogether; how could you? You simply need to build a healthy habit of moving more throughout the day, with occasional sitting stops. Start small: have a talk with your couch, your office chair, your car, your dining room chair. Note what keeps you on the couch, in your office chair, in your car. Find out what the barriers are to changing the habit of sitting, the barriers that keep you trapped in a sitting mode.

I asked myself why I sat in my easy chair to write this book. I answered that I liked the view I had out the window, an inspiring view. It always helped me get started and get over humps in my writing. Once the words flowed, I didn't need the view. I also admitted that I liked the comfort of my easy chair, the way it held me while I worked on a difficult task. I like to relax after being physically active, which happens many times in my day. Sitting in the chair was my respite while I got some brainwork done. Those were my excuses, my barriers to changing the sitting habit when I write.

Since my sitting time expands when I am working on a particular project, I struggle with getting in enough physical activity during intense sessions of composition. So to "walk" the talk of this chapter, I made myself get up out of my chair, stroll around, look out the window, and stretch my back. Then I decided to be extra adventurous and placed my laptop on the higher end of the kitchen island where I could stand and type at the same time. As I typed, I wiggled, I stretched, I breathed more deeply.

The words flowed, and I accomplished my daily quota with special ease. I wasn't reaching for snacks to keep me going, I wasn't slurping sugary drinks to wake up my brain. I was alert and focused while standing. Now when I need inspiration, I go stand in front of the window and/or listen to some music.

You too can break a barrier that keeps you sitting. Pick one of those habitual barriers and experiment with alternatives. Instead of turning on the television to watch a show to unwind when you get home from work or errands, put on your walking shoes and check out the landscaping while walking around your neighborhood.

Figure out what needs your habitual sitting meets. Sitting is an absolute necessity only if you are fainting and can't stand up, or if you're in excruciating pain that can be eased only with sitting. When you locate the need, make a note of it, and start a change journal. Keep this up for 30 days. Every time you come up against the barrier, ask yourself what you need and resolve it by taking care of your need and then move back to the nonsitting activity. Now when I need to rest awhile after being active, I sit for half an hour, until I'm no longer tired. Then I get up and find a different position in which I can write.

It takes a commitment to adopt the walking life. As with changing any habit, start small. Here are suggestions to turn on your "activity switch." Note where and when you can fit walking into your life. Ask yourself, as you leave your house why you need to drive to do what you are about to do. Note your reason. Is it a time constraint? Is it weather? Is it that you have to carry stuff? Soon enough, you will give yourself an extra 10 minutes, find that umbrella or warm coat, get a backpack to carry things. You'll be walking to the market if you are lucky enough to have one nearby. Ask yourself as you sit in your office, what your alternatives are. Can you stand and work on your computer? Can you pace your office while talking on the phone? Can you invite work partners for a "walk and talk" meeting? Before you know it, you'll be walking two miles while at work.

Each little walk spurs your cells to regenerate—even a walk around your living room. Dr. Joan Vernikos, a NASA scientist, who studied the effect of being weightless on aging, tells us that we need to activate the G-force, the force of gravity, in our body every 30 minutes (be upright) to be healthy and live a long life. Instead of adding new clothes or new shoes to your life to make yourself feel better, get up, walk around, and add new healthy cells. They are free.

When you add walking to your life, even if it's just to pick up the mail at the end of a long driveway, it will give you a sense of purpose, a road to feeling more alive and to living lighter on the planet. It will also inspire you to tune in to the world around you.

As a woman past 50, your purpose isn't raising a family or taking care of those around you. In this phase of life, you can turn your attention back to yourself and find different purpose. Filled with the experiences and insights gleaned from your youth, you can reexamine your place in the world and let creativity infuse your living. Exploring unknown pathways, both literally and figuratively, can become your new goal.

The act of walking can give you back your confidence. When you walk, you'll experience balance as well as physical and mental joy, and you'll discover that you can walk yourself to health and renewed wellbeing.

6 Ways to Add Walking to Your Life
1. Stand more (set a timer and stand hourly, let your smartwatch or Fitbit alert you)
2. Change from playing video games to activity-promoting games such as geo-caching or buy an exercise video
3. Walk while talking on the phone

4. Get a pedometer and count your steps—increase your steps from your baseline

5. Take stairs up one floor or down two (consider more) when you're in a building with a stairwell

6. Park your car in the farthest corner of the parking lot and walk to your destination

6: Walk! Your Life Depends on It

She was a salesperson—a good one. She traveled 300 days a year selling books to school districts. She lived in hotel rooms, ate in restaurants, drove in rental cars. She made good money, and at her age, she needed it to catch up from a life of raising kids as a single mother, barely getting by, and collecting debt instead of wealth. She had taken the opportunity when her last son was in high school to venture out on the corporate sales road. By the time she was 60, she had a stimulating job, she could see a retirement fund in her future, and her kids were well on their way to success. Life looked good. All she needed was a place to call home, a place where she could live out her days.

And then it hit her. She started having trouble sleeping and her mood plummeted, a mood that couldn't be lifted by drinking sugary soda. Her usual upbeat spirit dissipated. She tried more work and earned more success, but her body didn't enjoy it. Post-menopausal weight gain put her on the road to a heart attack, or type 2 diabetes, or both.

She was a smart woman. She knew the facts. She had seen *Food, Inc.* and *Supersize Me*, which gave her food for thought. So she made one change: she cut out the soda and replaced it with diet soda. After 6 months, the diet soda went by the wayside, and water took its place. Her meals became smaller, lighter. Her weight didn't go down much. She knew she had to exercise. But how and when? Hotel gyms were small unattractive places, and there wasn't time and consistency enough in her life to join a gym or attend a class.

She started walking: 1 mile a day, 2 miles a day, from her hotel. Then she walked while making phone calls, pacing in her suite. She decided she would get a Fitbit, count her steps and work up to 5 miles a day. Walking became her companion, her new goal in life.

After 18 months she had lost 50 pounds and logged 6000 miles of walking—in other words, twice across the USA! She stood at her desk, she paced while making deals, she stood and walked while training clients, she walked every morning from her hotel to find some piece of receptive earth. Her mood was upbeat, and she started sleeping well again.

By walking, she had taken her life back.

7: For the Love of Nature

I walked in nature because I found connectedness there, a sense of belonging I craved in the world of humans and rarely found.

My experiences in nature as a child were limited to beach life; there were occasional visits to man-made forests, but the beach gave me a sense of openness, the greatness beyond me and my small world, the unknown. The spaciousness opened my heart while the endless, rhythmic water enveloped me and taught me the comfort of being held as well as the danger of its powerful force. The wind—there always *was* wind in Holland—was something to forge against. It developed the muscles in my legs as I bicycled into it, leaning on the handlebars, or walked, head bent, coat flapping. For my young-adult emotional love affairs, the beach became my go-to place to walk off a heartache or untangle a knotty situation. Walking in nature became therapeutic.

When I ended up on the west coast of the United States in my twenties, I lived out in the country. Country life brought much physical work from cutting firewood to turning compost piles to building shelters. To relax from hard work and stretch my body in easy movement, it seemed natural to go for a walk. But walking in the country wasn't as easy as Henry David Thoreau described it in New England 1862:

> I can easily walk ten, fifteen, twenty, any number of miles, commencing at my own door, without going by any house, without crossing a road except where the fox and the mink do: first along by the river, and then the brook, and then the meadow and the wood-side. There are square miles in my vicinity which have no inhabitant.

On my hikes, I had to cross fields and woods that belonged to someone; they were often fenced off, with or without NO TRESPASSING signs. No longer are there accessible square miles that aren't owned by individuals in our overpopulated world unless we go to a designated wilderness. Living in the country, I found that I had to walk on roads to avoid charging dogs, animal traps, and defensive gun owners. So we ended up moving to a small town with easy public access to the natural world.

To experience the therapeutic value of walking in nature, you have to find a park, riverfront, woods, beach, or hills with public access and maintained trails. Times have changed since Thoreau wrote his essay "Walking," for what he described has come to pass:

> But possibly the day will come when it will be partitioned off into so-called pleasure-grounds, in which a few will take a narrow and exclusive pleasure only,—-when fences shall be multiplied, and man-traps and other engines invented to confine men to the public road and walking

on God's earth shall be construed to mean trespassing on some gentleman's grounds. To enjoy a thing exclusively is commonly to exclude yourself from the true enjoyment of it. Let us improve our opportunities, then, before the evil days come.

The "evil days" as Thoreau calls them are the times we live in. The exclusive enjoyment of individual property now prevents others from enjoying the land. If we want to walk cross-country, we must seek a designated wilderness. I will discuss that more later in the book.

Walking in a natural setting has a therapeutic effect on your mind *and* on your body. The softer terrain of woodland trails, sandy beach, and grassy paths allows for an easy landing with each step, a natural, more flowing movement through your spine. The unevenness of the terrain will exercise the smaller muscles in your feet and legs, making you more flexible. It will force you to work more with your body's balancing system and strengthen it, always a plus after age 50.

When I take a 5-mile walk on hard surfaces, sidewalks, or roads, my back aches after 45 minutes. When I walk on a dirt trail, my back is fine. Choose your walks as wisely as you can. Your body will thank you for it.

Planning Your Walk.

Few of us have the time and inclination to go out as Thoreau did: he set off on a walk and let his impulse and curiosity take him wherever they led. Before you plan out your walks too much, however, you might consider Thoreau's writing and find that, despite the old-fashioned language he uses, the art of walking is more than knowing where to go and what to wear.

I have met with but one or two persons in the course of my life who understood the art of Walking, that is, of taking walks—who had a genius, so to speak, for sauntering, which word is beautifully derived "from idle people who roved about the country, in the Middle Ages, and asked charity, under pretense of going à la Sainte Terre," to the Holy Land, till the children exclaimed, 'There goes a Sainte-Terrer,' a Saunterer, a Holy-Lander.

They who never go to the Holy Land in their walks, as they pretend, are indeed mere idlers and vagabonds; but they who do go there are saunterers in the good sense, such as I mean. Some, however, would derive the word from sans terre without land or a home, which, therefore, in the good sense, will mean, having no particular home, but equally at home everywhere. For this is the secret of successful sauntering.

My father was a saunterer. Once when he visited me from the old country, he looked out my window to the mountains across the valley and said, his voice trailing off, "I wonder how long it will take to walk to those mountains. I think I'll find out."

He made himself a sandwich and took off, choosing roads and paths in the general direction he wanted to go. He was gone most of the day. When he finally came back, he hadn't reached the mountains he saw out of my window. "It's a lot farther than I thought," he said. "There is a valley beyond each ridge, and you have to climb up and down to get to the next one." Coming from the flat lands he had "sauntered" into new territory. He had discovered, been unsure, and made decisions. He had learned about the land and made it his own. He was satisfied with his day of walking.

Turning your daily walks into sauntering can add mindfulness to your walks. You'll walk with your senses and you'll become an active and aware part of your environment. As Thoreau wrote in *Walden,* "Not till we are lost, in other words, not till we have lost the world, do we begin to find ourselves, and realize where we are and the infinite extent of our relations." What could be better?

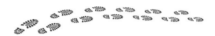

Not till we are lost, in other words, not till we have lost the world, do we begin to find ourselves.

8: Walking and Travel

There was a joke in my family about our vacations: Dad would go out to find a place to buy newspapers, and he wouldn't show back up at the hotel for at least 2 hours. He never failed to lose his way as he explored new territory, for my dad was a saunterer, as I've said, a curious man who thought he didn't need a map or advice from others. His curiosity led him to new places while my mother waited anxiously for his return. Just when she'd reached the end of her composure, he'd show up, glowing with information and discovery.

The wanderer trait must run in our family. The story goes that my grandfather at age 78, while on vacation with a group in Germany, went for a walk in the Schwarzwald, the Black Forest, lost his way, and spent the night in the woods without ill effects. I recognize the trait in myself. When I visit with family, I go for walks and lose my way trying to find new and interesting routes. Making it back at an agreed-upon time has proved difficult when I've found yet another nice trail in the woods that goes in the general direction of my daughter's house. However, wandering my way around the concrete jungle of Scottsdale, Arizona, as the temperatures rose to 110 degrees, turned out to be no joke. My "just going for a little walk" now gets this response: "Take your phone with you, so we can come get you if you get lost."

I do end up going farther than I planned, then have to find a route back that may not always cut through the neighborhoods in a way I hoped. But I never think of it as getting lost.

When you become a walker, travel needn't stop you from walking. Traveling to unfamiliar places offers an opportunity to explore on foot, to sharpen your senses, to discover the unknown.

Walking While in Transit

Airports offer great opportunities to get a walk between long periods of sitting. If at all possible, I walk from my arrival gate to my next departure gate. Years ago, however, when the Detroit airport had its major overhaul and sported a nice long walking corridor, I decided I would just get to my next gate on foot. It couldn't be that far! I was wrong. I ended up walk/running for 25 minutes to catch my flight, my carry-on roller in tow.

I've learned my lesson. I get to my next gate as soon as I can, and then assess the time I have left to take a walk. Further, when you get to your destination, you might walk off the tired travel feeling by heading to your ground transportation on foot. If possible, take public transportation into the city, get off a stop before your destination, and walk the rest of the way.

If you travel by car, use rest stops to walk. Your body (and mind) will thank you, and feeling more alive when you arrive is well worth the extra time. I figure in an extra half hour for a 6-hour car trip, giving myself 2 or 3 stops.

Few of us travel by boat anymore, but if you're lucky enough to do so, you might find yourself limited in your movements. The decks of cruise ships offer some walking opportunities, but the sailboats I've been on put a cramp in my walking lifestyle. Sailing the gorgeous Caribbean was wonderful, but walking on a hot, humid, bug-infested island and crawling through thick brush turned out to be more a chore than a pleasure. I write those walks off as "experiences."

Walking at a Destination Point

Once you arrive at your destination, figure out what your walking opportunities are. If you're visiting with family or friends, tell them about your new practice of walking and invite them along to show you the sights. It will be safer and more relaxing to have someone along who knows the territory. Don't let unwilling hosts stop you from walking, though; get a local map and figure out a route to explore. As a visiting grandma, I find that I have to take the initiative if I'm going to accelerate the grandbaby pace and get the walks I need. Others aren't going to organize them for me. Often it's a relief to get away by yourself for a while when visiting, and it offers a break for your hosts. They can attend to some of their own business while you're occupied on your walk.

When traveling as a tourist, you can easily incorporate walking to museums, historical sites, or parks. Join a walking tour; many cities now offer them. They are fun and informative and will keep you moving. Many tours incorporate daily walking: they're called active vacations.

One of my rowing buddies, an avid foreign traveler, told me recently that her experience of a tour I organized for rowers changed her concept of travel completely as she rowed or biked from small town to small town in Holland. Exercise was no longer confined to certain times of the week in a specified location; it had become a way of spending her days, at home and abroad. "From now on I only want active vacations," she declared.

When traveling for business, arrange your day as you would a working day at home. Make time for your walk, either in the workout room of the hotel (my least favorite place) or outside. Ask the hotel management for nearby parks or other walking opportunities. If you get one or two walks in on a busy work/travel day, your focus will be sharper and you'll make better business decisions.

When traveling, take the safety precautions described at the end of the next chapter, and take extra precautions when you are traveling in a foreign culture. You might stand out as a tourist, a stranger, because of your looks, and you'll be more of a target for pickpockets and potential harassers. Do your research on safety considerations for the place you're traveling to. Big western cities often carry more risks than a remote village in a developing country. I feel less safe walking in Barcelona than in the countryside around Sarnath, the Buddha's place of study in India. I take my precautions and walk when and where I can.

As a walking woman, it helps to travel light. Wear your walking shoes on the plane and pack just one other comfortable pair of shoes in your suitcase. Bring or wear protective clothing, and rain and sun gear where needed. Leave the multiple clothing changes at home; you can wear them again when you get back. Suitcases load you down and stop you from walking en route. Challenge yourself and fit what you need into a carry-on case; it will save you money and time, and enable you to walk. I've gone to warm Mumbai and cold Amsterdam in a single trip and managed to squeeze my down jacket, hat, gloves, warm sweater, and pants into a carry-on case along with my lighter, tropical clothing. Layers of clothing and a down jacket that fits in its own pocket were the key. Lightweight backpacking clothing, such as a pair of stretchy, easy-to-wash hiking pants that look decent enough for dining out, can double as travel clothing.

Walking from Place to Place

Women have walked across entire countries. Some have walked for a cause, some for the experience. To become a walking woman, you don't need to walk long distances. You become a walking woman when you make the commitment to walk when possible, to choose walking over the easy way of transporting yourself: the car.

If you become a walking woman, reward yourself at some point with a walking vacation. Europe offers splendid opportunities for walking from place to place carrying a light backpack while a host transports your luggage to your next lodging. Many European countries, where distances between places are short, offer organized walking tours.

If you're adventurous and want to cut costs, you can put your own trip together. Imagine sleeping in the tartan-clad bedroom of a local sailors' hotel one night and a medieval castle another night, exploring old ruins along the way and having lunch in a pub while talking with locals about how they make the area brews, all the while using your legs and breathing the fresh air. Such are the delights awaiting you!

Contact local tourist organizations or use Google for maps of walking routes. These maps will provide you with lodging options on the way. You pick the distance you want to walk in a day and contact a bed-and-breakfast connected to the route. There are actually apps as well that allow you to follow walking routes and make your reservations as you walk.

Walking for a Cause

As I mentioned earlier, women have walked long distances for a cause. In a desperate attempt to save her family from losing their property, Helga Estby and her daughter walked (in long skirts!) across the USA in 1896 for a wager. They were the first women we know of to walk across the United States. You can read about their journey in the book *Bold Spirit* by Linda Lawrence Hunt. In the year 2000 at age 90, Granny D. walked across the United States for campaign finance reform.

Some women must walk for the cause of survival. Unknown pioneer women and Native American women have trekked long distances for food and shelter. Today many women in African and Asian countries still must walk long distances daily to get water, find food, or escape from violent tribal wars.

To support these unknown women, I organized a walk for a cause. I invited friends, some of them hesitant walkers, to walk with me daily for a week and raise money to support women in poverty and war-struck countries. We walked 5 miles daily, rain or shine, 10,000 steps a day, a distance many women and girls must walk to get their daily water. We raised more than a thousand dollars. The walkers felt better for their efforts and made new connections with other walking women. Several women turned the corner on adopting a walking lifestyle. I got my spring training in by carrying a loaded backpack. Walking for a cause became a win-win for all!

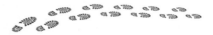

You become a walking woman when you make the commitment to walk when possible, to choose walking over the easy way of transporting yourself: the car.

Walking, then, becomes a lifestyle and no longer just a form of exercise. When you walk, you will experience the world around you with more sensory immediacy. You won't look at the world from behind glass, but rather feel, smell, hear, and absorb it at close hand. You will find community as you make a connection with people on your way with a nod, a hello, or a conversation.

9: Becoming an Active Walker

If you haven't been an active daily walker but want to become one, you're embarking on a change that will usher in a revolution, going against the grain of what you've been taught until now. Efficiency and ease drive our economy and drive our lives. Saving time is sacred. When you start walking, you give up ease and you give up timesaving efficiency. If you were raised on a diet of easy transportation, it will take a new mindset to incorporate walking into your life. Still, the long-term outcomes I've mentioned earlier in this book will be your gains: health, confidence, and a new outlook on living.

To begin walking sounds simple: put on your shoes and walk. It actually is that simple. The problems start when you don't know how far you can walk, when you can't find sidewalks or other safe places to walk, when you don't have shoes that are comfortable after a half mile of walking. The success of your newfound challenge depends on how much you walk, where you walk, and what you wear.

To get started, it's important to assess what your walking activity is at present. Get a tracking device you can wear on your wrist, or a pedometer, or use an app on your phone (newer phones have a built-in activity-tracking apps) that measures your steps as you go through your day. You may be surprised or shocked by the number you see at the end of a day. Are your numbers showing that you're leaning toward *sitting disease* or are they showing that you're on your way toward fitness and health?

If you're a sitter, make a list of tasks in your day you can do while standing or walking. Pick two of these sitting activities and walk while you do them. Let's say you sit to talk on the phone or to drink your morning cup of coffee or tea; instead of sitting, walk around while you do these things. Your body will thank you. Do you answer your mail on your computer while sitting? Set up your computing device so you can stand while using it and answer your mail while standing and moving. Do you sit to read the paper? Plug into news via radio and podcasts and walk while listening. I haven't figured out how to walk and knit, but I *have* seen Tibetans walk and spin their wool in the Himalayas, so I'm sure there's a way if I put my mind to it. I want to remind you: walking versus sitting is a mind-set.

If your tracker surprises you, and you find yourself to be a "mover" during your day, you may be logging more miles than you know. If you add outside activities you can do while walking, such as getting groceries, doing errands, or visiting a friend. your daily miles will increase even more. If you use public transportation, walk to a bus stop farther away from your current point of departure or get off at a stop before your destination.

The current recommendation to support your health is to walk 10,000 steps a day, 4.6 miles. That number can be less, depending on what other physical activities you engage in. Without taking a formal "walk," I average 2–3 miles a day just doing what I need to do. Find out how much walking you're doing already!

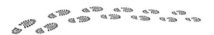

The long-term outcome of walking is health, confidence and a new outlook on living.

Fitting Walking into Your Life

At this point even if you haven't added walking as a separate activity to your life, you've just changed how you go about your daily business. Yes, it may take more time to get the errands done if you do them while walking, but you'll gain much more than just getting the errand out of the way, including not having to look for parking. I use my bike if I don't have the time to walk to complete my errands. That way I'm still moving my body.

If you have a job or responsibilities that keep you occupied most of your day, finding time to walk can be an issue. Starting small in ways I have mentioned will help you develop a walking mind-set. Once you integrate more walking into doing your errands or caring for a grandchild or an elder, it will be easier to take the next step and set a daily or weekly walking goal.

I learned of a woman who got into the habit of rising early to walk her dog before going to work. She liked the quiet of the early morning walk so much that she ended up walking two hours before getting ready for work, which included a 45-minute commute. Her evening walk with the dog easily took up an hour as well. Her schedule looked like this: rise at 4:00 a.m., walk till 6:15 a.m., get to work by 8:00 a.m., return home at 6:00 p.m., walk the dog till 7:00 p.m., make dinner and eat, and get to bed by 9:00 p.m. When I heard about her walking habit, she had been doing it for 20 years. By the way, she was happily married. You can see that there wasn't time for TV watching in her day. She had other priorities.

Walking with Aches and Pains

Do aches and pains stop you from walking? Do they stop you from going shopping, going out to dinner or a movie, or going on vacation? Do the aches and pains stop you from living your life, from doing the things you want to or need to do? Sadly, in our society, walking doesn't "walk" into your life; you have to want to do it to make it happen.

Older people heal more slowly than younger ones. Do you let this stop you from getting active again after an injury? Or does the lack of desire to walk stop you? As an older friend once said to me, "Don't ask me if it hurts when I walk. It hurts all the time. It's no different when I walk, so I'll just keep walking." This woman walks because she wants to, pain or not.

You don't necessarily have to walk with pain after 50. With some care you can let walking be your vehicle to feeling better. When my back acted up a few years ago every time I walked more than 45 minutes, I considered what to do. As soon as I stopped walking, the pain vanished. It was tempting to avoid a longer walk. But I already was so committed to walking that I followed my heart and explored what caused the pain, so I could get rid of it. I noticed that with a weight in my backpack the pain didn't occur. That told me it had something to do with my posture while I walked. It took a winter of visits to a doctor and physical therapist to find the cause. Eventually my osteopath ordered an MRI and found that I had a bulging disc in my mid-back. Stretches, exercise, and continued walking, especially the longer hikes with a backpack, have healed the injury over 2 summers. I can now go for an ordinary 1-hour walk without my back acting up. If I had stopped walking, I would not have found out what was going on and, risking other problems in the process, wouldn't have healed myself.

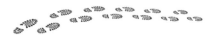

Don't let your age determine your healing! Let your mindset determine what you can and cannot do.

Young people assume that they will heal quickly. Older people not so much. Don't let your age determine your healing! Let your mindset determine what you can and cannot do. I walk with a knee that doesn't have much cartilage left; I wear an elastic support and do exercises to strengthen the muscles all around the knee. I keep swelling down and hike sometimes 18-20 miles a day without ill effect! My orthopedist said after diagnosing the problem, "Why do you need to hike 18 miles a day?" thus relegating me to a less active category. I responded, "Because I want to."

Another doctor told me, "Hike if you can control the pain. It will not create more rapid wear, and may slow it down."

When your knee doesn't work anymore, get a new knee!" I liked the way my doctor's attitude aligned with mine. I walk with my crooked back, my worn knee, and my developing bunions. I care for these aberrations as much as possible by adding special exercises and foot treatments to slow down the process of my aging, twisting, shrinking body. At this point, taking anti-inflammatory meds now and then are my go-to assists to keep me walking.

On the long-distance trail I hear young people complain about body pains. Their feet hurt, they have stress fractures, their backs go out, their muscles are sore, you name it. Aches and pains happen at any age. How we react to them differs. The young ones quit only if they're forced to do so. Often they wait much too long before they go into rest and healing mode. The older ones become hesitant to continue their activity. Neither approach is helpful for the body's healing. Listen to your body, stay active, encourage healing, and come back to walking as soon as possible without injuring yourself further. Walking will heal you. Your attitude will start the healing, or at least keep you living with gusto.

The Walking Route

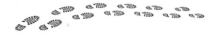

Start your walking life with walking around your home, your place of work, your neighborhood.

As you become a walker, you plan where to go each day to fit in your 5 miles. Maybe you develop a regular route and are happy completing it; maybe you do your errands and get your walking in. At some point you may look for variety in terrain or variety in view. You can take a road not taken before and see where it leads you.

You can start your walking life with walking around your home. You can walk at your place of work, the gym, your neighborhood, a nearby park, the hills, the beach, the forest, and along highways and rivers. It doesn't matter where you walk as long as you feel safe and the terrain isn't too difficult for you. Start small and increase your distance as the weeks go by. Walk your dog, if you have one, to give yourself a reason to go out.

Consider where you take your walk. For a short walk it makes little sense to get into a car and drive to a walking destination, but if your neighborhood doesn't offer decent walking opportunities, take yourself to a better place by car if you must. If possible, choose nature over concrete for your walk: it's easier on your body, and it will enhance your mood. Choose walking paths and sidewalks over roadsides; you will relax more if you don't have to watch out for traffic.

If you're an urban walker, choose a less busy neighborhood or a city park. Traffic and noise stress our bodies. If traffic and noise are unavoidable, plug into soothing music while still paying attention to your surroundings as you walk. Suburban walkers might want to find a park or waterway that breaks up the monotony of similar houses and streets. Country walkers often can't find sidewalks or walking paths and have to walk on narrow highways or roads. Make sure you face oncoming traffic when you walk on a highway, or pick unpaved roads, such as logging roads and wagon tracks where possible, so you can walk without having to jump away from passing cars. Many cities and small towns now have maps of walking trails and offer walking tours. Check online with your municipality for a map with ideas for walks.

10: Training a 50-Plus Body

To regularly walk 5 miles a day you have to train your body. Training is part of changing your body and mind, readying you for new experiences.

If you haven't been an exerciser, you might wonder if it's too late to get in shape for the walking life. The good news is that after 50, you can improve your fitness, one step at a time. Consistent training is crucial for the older body. It takes much longer to regain fitness at a more advanced age than when you're younger, so it's important to hang on to your gains. It's like building your financial independence: when you're young, you can afford losses because you'll have time to rebuild your nest egg; later in life it isn't easy to recover from those losses. This chapter will guide you through training to get you ready for your "walks gone wild."

Walking Pace

When you start out, walk at an easy pace without stressing your breathing. As you work up to longer distances, you can increase your pace, increase your heart rate, and work up a little sweat on warm days. (For more on this, see High-Intensity Interval Training later in this chapter.)

Warm-Up and Cool-Down

A warm-up for a walk can simply mean starting at an easy pace for the first 5 minutes to let your heart rate increase slowly. Cooling down can be a slower pace at the end of your walk during the last few minutes, depending on how far you're walking, and a few stretches when you get home or back to the office. The stretches will allow the blood to flow back from your muscles to the rest of your body, which helps remove lactic acid from your bloodstream, thus reducing soreness later.

Choosing a 0 to 5K Walking Program

With the current health trend to encourage people to walk more, many cities and municipalities offer 5K walking programs. You can usually find these programs online.

Below is an example of a 5K program. You can follow the steps suggested or create your own program. Keep in mind the importance of gradually increasing your activity and listening to your body.

Make sure to consult your physician if you have lived a sedentary life or have physical limitations or other health issues.

- Walk every day, 7 days a week. Increase your distance weekly; a half-mile increase is a reasonable goal
- Once you're up to 5 miles a day, keep walking 5 miles a day both by taking walks and walking while doing your activities. Wear a device that tracks your steps/miles.

0 TO 5 MI TRAINING SCHEDULE					
week 1	week 2	week 3	week 4	week 5	week 6
walk daily, start with 1/2 mi, work up to 1 mi	walk daily, start with 1 mi, work up to 1 1/2 mi	walk daily, start with 1 1/2 mi, work up to 2 mi	work from 2 up to 3 mi at a stretch 5 days/wk	work from 3 up to 4 mi at a stretch 4 days/wk	work from 4 up to 5 mi at a stretch 4 days/wk
			2 days/wk mix your miles with intermittent walking activities	3 days/wk mix your miles with intermittent walking activities	3 days/wk mix your miles with intermittent walking activities

High-Intensity Interval Training

The American Heart Association and other organizations have recommended for years that people complete 30 minutes or more of continuous, moderate-intensity exercise, such as a brisk walk, 5 times a week for overall good health. But now evidence shows that high-intensity interval walking has even better effects on health, especially on hypoglycemia and type 2 diabetes, on cardiac disease, and on mild-to-moderate Parkinson's symptoms.

When people hear about high-intensity interval training (HIIT), they envision athletes working hard to improve their time, to get an edge on their fitness. But you can pursue HIIT in many ways and on many levels. You can design your own workout or use an example below, to get started.

A Danish HIIT study compared HIIT with regular walking and found that people who had trouble sticking with an exercise routine were sticking with the HIIT because it was shorter (20 minutes, 3 times a week) and the variety in pace was more engaging.

HIIT is a 20-minute aerobic routine, such as walking, biking, running, or rowing. After a 5-minute warmup, the exerciser walks (or runs, bikes, and so on), ideally for 1 minute at 80 or 90 percent of her maximum heart rate (subtract your age from 220 and you will have your maximum heart rate), then spends 1 minute of recovery doing the same activity at an easy pace. The main objective is to alternate a high rate and a low rate. Repeat the effort and recovery segments 10 times for 20 minutes. You can check your heart rate by checking your pulse on the inside of your wrist: rest two fingers gently on the artery near the mound of the thumb as you walk or run (you must go into a run or fast walk to bring up your heart rate), count the pulse beats for 10 seconds, and multiply by 6 to get your heart rate. Even if you can't get your heart rate to 80 percent of its maximum, just creating a higher rate for 1 minute followed by an easy pace will be effective for starters.

In a group of middle-aged unfit people and a group of middle-aged cardiac patients, researchers found that despite the small time commitment required by this modified HIIT program, both the unfit volunteers and the cardiac patients showed significant improvements in their health and fitness after several weeks of practice.

Scientists noted other benefits in earlier studies. In unfit but otherwise healthy middle-aged adults, two weeks of modified HIIT training prompted the creation of far more cellular proteins involved in energy production and oxygen. The training improved the volunteers' insulin sensitivity and blood sugar regulation, lowering their risk of developing type-2 diabetes. Since then, scientists have completed a small, follow-up experiment involving people with full-blown type-2 diabetes. They found that even a single bout of the 1-minute hard, 1-minute easy HIIT training, repeated 10 times, improved blood sugar regulation throughout the following day, especially after meals.

HIIT training is not ideal or necessary for everyone. Martin Gibala, a professor of kinesiology at McMaster University in Ontario, Canada, who oversaw these high-intensity studies, noted, "If you have time for regular 30-minute or longer endurance exercise training then, by all means, keep it up. There's an impressive body of science showing that such workouts are very effective at improving health and fitness."

If you want to improve your health through walking and have limited time, include interval walking. If you do well with and prefer moderate-tempo regular walking, do that. In either case the result will be better health.

The 20-Minute HIIT Walk Workout

Below is an example of the HIIT workout for a treadmill where you can program your walking speed. Check your heart rate as you change your speed and hold on! Remember, this is an example, and the speed can be adjusted to suit your ability.

Using these examples of training schedules, you should get a good idea of how to shape your walking life. Take as long as you want to get to 5 miles a day, and let your physical or time constraints dictate your walking schedule. The 6-week training schedule is just a guideline. The important thing is that you walk more than you have been walking. If you've been on the couch too much, allow yourself a year to get your walking fitness in order. Once you achieve this, you might find yourself dreaming of bigger things.

HIIT							
warm-up	fast walk/jog	sprint	fast walk/jog	sprint	fast walk/jog	sprint	cool down
5 min at 3.5 speed	2 min at 4.0 mi speed	1 min at 6.0 mi speed	2 min at 4.0 mi speed	1 min at 6.0 mi speed	2 min at 4.0 speed	1 min at 6.0 speed	4 min at 3.5 speed

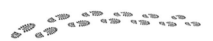

Take as long as you need to get to 5 miles a day. The important thing is that you walk more than you have been walking.

11: Walking Gear, Food and Safety

You don't need fancy sports clothing to walk, hike, or backpack. Clothing designed for being active and designed to protect you from exposure to the elements can enhance the experience.

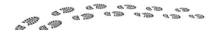

The most important piece of gear for walking is a good pair of shoes.

Walking Shoes

Whether you walk outdoors or indoors at a gym or in a mall, you need shoes. Walking shoes, hiking shoes, and running shoes: even though all of them cover your feet, they differ in how they function on the road or trail. You can wear any of them and walk, but why not choose a pair of shoes that is intended for your specific walking activity?

To choose walking shoes, consider the terrain, the strength of your feet or lack thereof, and the way your foot moves when you walk. Are you a supinator or a pronator (does your foot roll outward or inward as you walk) or are you in between? To find out, check the soles of shoes you've been wearing.

If the heel is worn down on the outside, you're a pronator; if it's worn down on the inside, you're a supinator; and if the heel wear is even, you're in between.

If you are a supinator, look for motion-control shoes; if you're a pronator, look for a neutral, cushioned shoe with maximum flexibility. If you're in between, you'll do best with a stability shoe with moderate flexibility.

Do you have high, low, or medium arches? If you don't know, step on a piece of colored paper—a brown paper bag will do—with wet feet and make an imprint of the sole of your foot. The narrower the imprint of the arching part of your foot is on the paper, the higher your arch is. You can have your feet assessed by a podiatrist (a foot specialist) if you have problem feet, so you can make an informed choice in shoe wear. If you have never experienced foot problems, you can choose your shoes by feel. If your feet and legs hurt after walking in them, you have the wrong shoes.

When choosing a walking shoe, consider the following:

Shape and flexibility. The best shoes for walking will have low, rounded heels that support the natural heel strike of a walker. As a test, bend a walking shoe while holding the heel in your hand. The shoe should bend where your toes naturally bend. The shoe should have some stiffness in the middle (unlike running shoes which need to flex more). A stiff last (the mold upon which the shoe is constructed) is more comfortable on rough terrain, such as a rocky mountain trail.

Arch support and footbed. A healthy foot needs little more than protection from wet, cold, rough terrain and support in the arch. A trend of barefoot running and walking erupted a decade ago, encouraging people to go back to a more native lifestyle, touting the health of walking barefoot. This way of moving was a positive experience for some, but many people ended up with unwanted injuries, such as inflamed tendons, painful arches, or stress fractures.

Although cushioned soles feel nice to sensitive feet, they don't help your feet get stronger. A very flexible shoe with a thin sole gives your foot a workout but will tire you more. Choose how much support you need for your foot based on the shape and strength of your feet.

Weight of the shoe. As you become a stronger walker, your shoe wear matters less, except for the weight of the shoe and the stiffness of the last (see above). A lighter shoe is easier on your legs since you'll be lifting less with each step. Choose a shoe with your walking goal in mind. You may end up with town/city walking shoes and country/forest terrain walking shoes.

There are resources online for choosing your walking shoes, such as http://www.the-fitness-walking-guide.com/womens-walking-shoes.html, or you can consult a podiatrist.

Whatever shoe you choose, make sure it fits well. When you become a walking woman, your foot will lengthen and widen, as it does with age, so buy your shoes bigger and leave room for expansion. It is painful to develop a neuroma, an inflamed nerve ending in and under the toe, from shoes that are too small. This will set you back in your walking goals. To get a good fit, I recommend buying your shoes later in the day after your feet have expanded from the day's walking.

You may already have shoes that will work for your walk. Buy new ones if the shoes you have show a series of fine cracks in the cushy part of the sole. You can see the cracks by looking at the sides of the soles of your shoes. The cracks show that the sole is breaking down. You can still walk in them, but they won't give you the support you want. I usually relegate my "old" but still wearable shoes to work around the garden or some other dirty nonwalking task.

Now that you have chosen your walking shoes, you're ready to go for a walk.

Food and Walking

Since walking is seen as a way to lose weight, eating is not the first thing we think of when we go walking. To prepare yourself for walking, though, make sure you have the energy to complete your walk. If you need a snack before you exercise, by all means eat something. If you're an early morning exerciser/walker, however, you may want to wait till you get back home before you eat.

If you walk in the evening, do it before you have dinner. Walking on a full stomach is not nearly as pleasant as walking with a lightly filled stomach. Once you establish a regular walking routine of at least 9 miles a week, your basal metabolism will burn food at a higher rate, so don't be surprised if your appetite increases. Eat healthful foods as needed, and your body will burn the calories.

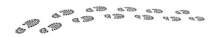

When you establish a regular walking routine, your basal metabolism will burn food at a higher rate.

Safety While Walking

If you're a low-mileage walker, you probably think little of danger when walking, at least not beyond watchfulness when crossing a street or choosing a safe neighborhood. Let your safety concerns be about visibility, traffic, and location. Reflective clothing makes you more visible to moving traffic. Take a tip from traffic safety and wear orange, yellow, or red, making you visible in all types of weather. If you can, choose the time of day of your walk so you can avoid high traffic times and walk in daylight.

If you work long hours at a job, you may walk in the early mornings or evenings in the dark or dusk. Again, a high-visability jacket or vest, or clothing with reflective stripes will let you stand out against traffic. If you walk in a dark area with little or no traffic, you expose yourself to the unknown, whether people or animals. Carry a whistle or other noisemaker to scare the person or animal away, or carry pepper spray. Don't plug in to your phone or iPod in those areas. You'll be less aware of what's going on around you.

To deter would-be attackers, avoid walking alone on the same route at the same time, day in, day out. Not only will you be safer, but the variety will enhance your enjoyment and lower your stress. Walking with someone else in a questionable environment at a questionable time of day will keep you safer. Besides, having a walking buddy can add to your enjoyment and the steadiness of your walking practice.

Section II

HIKING

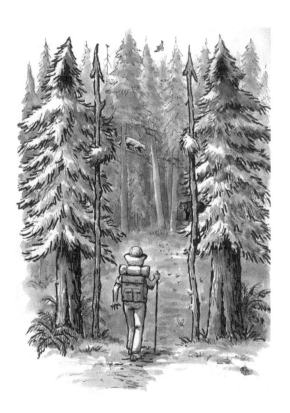

12: From Walking to Hiking

The word *hiking* evokes images of woods, mountains, and coastal areas with trails leading to craggy heights or hidden lakes. But even though we associate hiking with the wilderness, a hike is nothing more than a long walk taken to explore an area while carrying water, food, and basic survival essentials. If you are a walker—whether urban, suburban, country, or town—and feel at home with your new activity, you may feel the urge to take your walking further. The seasonal changes pull us outside, invite us to smell the woods, climb the hills, breathe the ocean air, and generally let us appreciate the vistas of the place we're exploring close to home or farther away.

If you've been managing your daily walks and you want to hike, all you have to do is explore on a bigger scale: pick a destination, follow a trail, or explore your environment farther from home on a day hike. Taking a hike doesn't mean you have to find the wilderness. You can hike the city. Dan Koeppel introduced the concept of urban hiking in 2004 when he detailed his preparation for mountain climbing by taking to the stairs in his neighborhood in Los Angeles. Laurel Leicht describes the development of urban hiking, now practiced in many big cities by hikers who may hike as much as 20 to 30 miles, take the stairs wherever they can to connect to cross roads, never walk the same street twice, bring a light pack, and even stay overnight to continue their hike the next day. PacSafe, a company that sells backpacks, lists on their blog the 10 best urban hiking cities, naming New York, Atlanta, Phoenix, and many West Coast cities. If you live in a city and the woods aren't within easy reach, you can still hike and find adventure doing so.

I live in a small town and can hike from home along the railroad tracks, across the boulevard, and up a steep street to the hills bordering the town where trails among the trees take me up and down, presenting views of the whole valley. Then I can circle back to the park that leads to downtown and home, a distance of nearly 10 miles. This hike is enough of a workout that I enjoy putting my feet up afterward, with a smile induced by endorphins and gratitude for a body that can take me places.

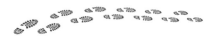

A satisfying hike done alone or with a friend becomes a therapeutic intervention against loneliness and many forms of stress.

A hike leaves the brain stimulated by surprising sights, smells, and sounds. The musty damp smell of leaves after the rain tells of our fertile earth in process. The crackling, honeyed smell of sun-dried grasses reminds us of the seeds blown by the wind to find that fertile soil. The gurgling of a little creek invites critters and people to quench their thirst. And even an urban hike can make us stand in amazement as thousands of bees swarm and buzz in a crab-apple tree in bloom, as warm stone steps lead you to a blue sky overlooking a river. Perhaps a bridge over a train yard presents you with the clanking music of cars hooking and unhooking. Surprises lurk everywhere if you take the time to walk out to meet them.

When I visited Boston, I "hiked" the 2.5-mile Freedom Trail and learned about Boston's history through my senses. I remember the elation when feeling the old cobblestones under my feet where men and women had walked and asked for shelter from persecution.

As I touched the tall brick houses along narrow streets, I imagined a world of craftsmen, schoolteachers, and entrepreneurs long ago; by sitting in the pews of the Old South Meeting House, I imagined overhearing the first democratic discussions about government.

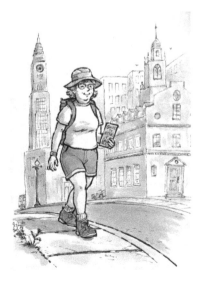

A hike then, is the surrender to the singular activity of moving your body for a period with no particular goal except to be outside taking in your environment. Hikes can be historical, natural, futuristic, or otherworldly. A night hike I took by the light of a full moon across endless lava deposits transported me to an imagined moonscape.

When we go on a hike, we tap into our deepest DNA. We touch the original intuitions and forces that drove us as humans to find food and shelter, to explore new places that could enable our tribe to survive. Remember, walking is embedded in our DNA. Hiking extends that walking activity and will make us more whole as human beings, no matter what age we are.

Trail Musings

I'm following a trail, wondering how the first people chose the way. The ones who went before me, the first ones, were the brave ones. They stepped out of ordinary life; they met the natural world full on, like a swimmer crossing a sea, not knowing how high the waves might be, how much the currents would pull.

The first ones looked far to the other side. They looked at the landmark ahead and picked a point to draw a course. The first ones answered the call of the land.

I planned this hike on the back of the brave ones, the scouts, the explorers. Without them going before me, I would not have my GPS, my compass, my maps, and pages from a guidebook.

I thank the first ones, the brave ones, with each step I take. I thank them for each sign I meet that tells me where I'm going and how far it is to where I want to go.

I'm not a risk-taker. I plan before I take off. I want to enjoy my hike in the wilderness without having to worry about finding the trail.

One day I lost the trail. I wasn't lost in the wilderness crisscrossing the forest. I just ended up on an unpaved road. It was mid-morning, and until noon I walked on this road, going in the southern direction I needed to go. Cars, mostly coming toward me, were slowing down as they approached. People were waving at me. I was having an inverse celebrity experience; I was the one being watched while doing the walking, while the audience was doing the riding. When I found an access point to the trail again, I was glad to get back on it. I was becoming shy of people, and solitude had its grip on me.

13: Planning Your Hike

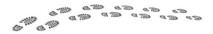

The best physical exercise to get in shape for hiking is walking. Walking is slow, methodical, repetitive, and low-impact, and anyone can do it.

A hike begins with a wish to get out, to escape your daily routine, to leave, temporarily, the people with whom you live. You may end up going with others who have the same inclination; you may go alone.

Thoreau was in the habit of starting a hike right out of his cabin door, but he lived in a time when he could find a country road, across meadows and fields, without having to pass through fences or ignore NO TRESPASSING signs. Few nowadays are lucky enough to access a trail into the woods his way.

If you live in a city, you can drive out to the country, the woods, the mountains, or the river's edge to hike in nature.

You can also walk out your door and hike the city. If you want to try the latter, get a city map and mark areas you don't know yet, those containing a park or other nature area; then scan the streets and figure out which ones might have less traffic. Plan an approximate route, noting where arterial streets interconnect. Once you have a distance mapped out, you can weave in and out of the arterial streets to discover what hides in the side streets, the cul-de-sacs, under bridges, and along waterways.

A different way to plan your urban hike is to pick one or two points of interest, such as buildings or public places you want to know more about, and plan a route connecting those points. Look up information on the building or the public place and create your own tour without stopping along the way. City walking tours fall more in the category of walks and have too many points of interest to allow you to get into the hiking mode of moving your body along a trail.

Whether you live in a big city, a small town, or the country, you can find hikes that will take you further into nature. Check with your local chamber of commerce and park organizations to find designated trails. You can get a local hiking book or go online to a hiking site to find the same information.

If you plan to leave your city or town to hike, find a hiking book that covers the place you want to visit or an online hiking directory that can help you find a trail that suits you. A good hiking directory should tell you the length of a trail; the difficulty factor of the trail, including elevations, directions to the trailhead; and the availability of water. It will mention interesting sights and vistas and give you your choice for the day of a long or short, difficult or easy outing.

Have fun: plan a hike, call a friend, and go out into the unknown.

Outfitting Yourself for Your Hike

Hiking Shoes

Walking shoes will do for most hikes up to 5 miles. If you plan a hike in mountainous terrain, you might want hiking shoes.

Hiking shoes and boots are all about disaster avoidance. Try stepping from algae-covered rock to algae-covered rock in a fast-running mountain stream, and you'll know what I'm talking about! Hiking miles on a lava-rock trail will massage your feet to the point of painful sensitivity if you don't have enough tread and stiffness protecting them. For most hikes, any shoe with a treaded, high-grip outsole will do. I can even wear my Teva sandals with treaded soles for easy hikes and be fine, but for more rugged terrain you'll want to invest in something more substantial to protect your feet and prevent ankle sprains and sore feet afterward. On rough terrain, the stiffer sole saves you from painful calves and feet.

The high-cut hiking boot is going out of fashion for long-distance hiking because of its weight—every step you take, you carry 5 pounds on your feet—but there is still a place for the boot among hiking footwear. Wear them when climbing mountains with rocky trails or when walking through wet or snowy conditions. Keeping your feet protected and dry trumps lightness.

I've met women who hike with the Vibram-soled five-fingered shoe or ultralight cover for their feet. They maintain that going almost barefoot changes their way of walking and makes their bodies stronger and healthier. If you're not used to this type of footwear in normal walking, I wouldn't recommend hiking with it.

You, the hiker, are the best judge of which shoe is best for you. Shoes are a highly individual commodity. As we age, our feet become more sensitive and we lose the cushioning under the balls of our feet.

It's worth trying out different styles and seeing how a particular shoe affects your overall bodily comfort. Outdoor Gearlab (outdoorgearlab.com) provides a review of hiking shoes and boots in terms of durability, fit, comfort, weight, and specificity of use. Check that out before you go shopping, so you'll know what you're looking for amid the great variety of hiking shoes.

Hiking Poles

Walking/hiking poles help you on your hiking trail with both balance and speed. If you have problems walking, poles can be your support to get started. If you use your arms to pull yourself forward and up the incline with the poles, you'll give those underarm wattles a workout and make your stride steadier and stronger. Walking poles are an accepted item for the long-distance hiker for the reasons I mention here. They are not a telltale sign of a senior hiker.

Before you buy, try a pair borrowed from someone you know. Use two sticks if you don't want to spend the money. Walking poles don't have to be fancy to work for you. A warning for people with carpal tunnel syndrome: hiking poles aggravate your symptoms if you create too much stress on the wrist.

The Backpack

For a walk you may bring only a water bottle or a fanny pack to hold your keys and phone, but for a day hike you'll want a backpack to hold water, extra clothing, rain gear, food for the day, and your camera, map, compass, and so on. You may use a backpack you have lying around, but if you shop for a new daypack keep in mind what purpose the pack needs to serve. Are you going to climb over rocks, scaling mountainsides, or are you going to follow an established trail? Are you going to be hiking in summer only, or do you want to hike in shoulder seasons—early spring and late fall—when weather might be changeable, requiring more equipment?

As you develop your hiking ability, you will upgrade your pack occasionally. A small frame pack is easy on the shoulders and back. A tight-hugging climbing pack distributes the weight really well. Talk to an outdoor specialist when choosing a day pack; ask other hikers why they have the pack they carry; read the reviews. As with shoes, there are many choices in varying price ranges, and new products come out every year. If you read the spring gear issue of *Backpacker* magazine, you can make a more informed choice.

Hiking Clothes

Besides shoes, you'll need clothing that lets you move easily, isn't too heavy, and allows your body to breathe. Give yourself comfortable clothes that serve you when you're moving, perspiring, and going through temperature changes. For the fashionistas among us, I have good news: you can let yourself be attractive and practical at the same time. There's a plethora of slimming and colorful outdoor clothing available. The ingenuity of its design will make you appreciate that just-right zip-up level of your jacket when the wind blows, that thumbhole in the shirt to protect the mound of your hand when holding the hiking pole, and those side zippers in your sun shirt for when the temperatures rise and you're determined not to develop skin blisters. We've come a long way from the clammy, sweaty cotton T-shirts of the past.

Layered clothing allows for temperature changes both in your body and in the air. Temperature will determine what and how many layers you'll need. Make sure your pants or skirt—yes, hiking skirts exist and some people prefer the freedom a skirt provides—can stand up to a slide off a rock or a tangle with branches. Jeans can do the job for a day hike but are stiff and heavy, unless you have lightweight stretch jeans, and in that case are they still called "jeans"? Zip-off pants allow you to wear shorts when temperatures rise and the terrain is not full of brush or scratchy undergrowth. Long-sleeved (sun) shirts are a must if you value your skin. Ditto for a wide-brim hat to protect you from the sun's rays. Expect changes in the weather; carry extra clothing.

When you're out hiking, you can tell the older hikers from the younger ones not only by their face but also by their garb. Older hikers wear more protective clothing; the younger ones wear short shorts and tank tops. On one of my long hikes, I met up with a young woman and exchanged trail information. I said, "I'm glad to see you wearing sensible clothing for this trip. Most women your age I meet are exposing their skin on the trail."

She grinned and said, "I know. I'm doing my second through-hike" (she was hiking the length of the Pacific Crest

Trail, trying to break the record) "and I don't want skin cancer when I'm your age." I told her of meetings I'd had with other young hikers and how I'd been playing "mother" to them, warning them, and showing them what happens to skin when you've been getting too much sun. Our age difference fell away. Between her young woman and my crone we agreed that we wanted to enjoy the trail, at a different speed but in the same wearable fashion.

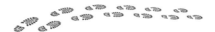

Even for a day hike, consider possible weather changes and bring an extra layer.

Hiking Food and Water

Food for day hiking needs to sustain you, be easy to carry, and offer reserves in case of unwanted delays. Always pack an extra bar or snack to carry you over in case of injury, inclement weather, or, God forbid, losing your way. Even though you can survive for days without food, it sure helps to have sustenance when you need to be alert and make life-saving decisions. For a day hike, any kind of food will do, from leftover pizza to sandwiches or trail mix.

A cucumber or other crisp veggie is a refreshing and nutritious snack when you've been climbing and sweating. A chocolate bar in cold weather can pick you right up. As we get older, our bodies function better with frequent small amounts of food, and that goes for hiking as well.

Bring drinking water or a water purifier to keep you hydrated for your hike, and some extra in case you are delayed or injured. Ask yourself how much you will sweat. Count on needing 1 liter for each 4 miles you hike on a summer day, more if it's an extremely hot day. Difficulty of the terrain will increase your water needs.

14: Staying Safe on Your Hike

Like walking, hiking is considered a safe activity. There are inherent dangers in many things we do, from driving a car to not exercising to hiking. That being said, the danger of hiking if you add it to the pool of risks in your everyday life is negligible—especially if you plan and prepare well. An important part of planning a hike is planning for a successful outcome. In Chapter 13 we discussed how to plan your itinerary, what to wear, and what to bring in terms of food and water. These preparations contribute to your safety on your hike. But even if you think you've covered all the bases, it doesn't take much to tip the scales from a pleasant hike to a dangerous situation. I still remember a day hike when I learned I need to overprepare, even when going on a seemingly innocuous day outing.

The day started sunny, and a hike around a well-known rock formation nearby in May seemed the perfect thing to do. A friend had told me of a new trail that connected partway up a well-known path to Pilot Rock with the PCT and then meandered in a wide arc around the rock. "Easy to follow," she said, "an 8-10-mile journey." I figured it would take us 4 hours at the most. With a friend I set out midday, expecting to be back at the car around 5:00 p.m. We followed the signs and the wide trail, circling around the rock formation: expansive views, wildflowers, and a pleasant temperature.

Around 4:30 p.m. we crossed a creek. The trail forked, and it wasn't clear which path to take to get back to the car. We traveled toward the rock formation and turned left. When the trail ended in dense brush and the rubble of downed trees, we backtracked and followed the old logging road in the other direction, figuring it would turn back toward the rocks and our car. As we walked on, we saw two women—who turned out to be researchers—working in the woods gathering data. We asked them if they knew how soon this trail would meet up with the PCT. They looked puzzled and asked if we had a map. We didn't because this trail had been built recently and we'd figured it wasn't on the map yet. The women told us we were heading in the wrong direction and offered to put a copy of their forestry map on my phone. It included a thin black line leading toward the PCT. They said as soon as they were finished working they would pack up and go in that direction to their parked truck.

We went ahead of them so they could catch up with us if we ran into trouble on the trail they had pointed out. We climbed over trees and struggled to find a noticeable trail. Then the trail clearly dead-ended. What to do? We sat down on a log and looked at our options. Nightfall was only 2 hours away, and we didn't have a tent or sleeping bag. We decided we should turn around and, if need be, walk back where we had come from, even if it would take us till midnight to get to our car. We hoped we would be lucky enough to meet up with the forestry women and follow them out. We did meet the women again and traipsed behind them while they used their GPS device to find their way out. Apparently the trail shown on the map had disappeared for lack of use. It started to rain; the going was up-hill through the forest. The women were young and strong and moved at a fast pace, but my companion and I were running on adrenaline. After an hour and a half, we arrived at their truck, drenched but safe. They gave us a ride to our car.

It was all too easy to see that we could have spent the night out in the woods, wet and cold, before help came or before we found our way out. Because of the rain, the moon wasn't giving any light, and hiking back would have been difficult. Cell phone reception was spotty, and it would have been difficult to signal our location to rescuers during the night. We had water and a little food, but not enough warm clothes for both of us. Making a fire would have been problematic in the rain.

To be better prepared for this hike, we would have needed an accurate map that showed us that the trail we had in mind was an 18-mile loop, not an afternoon hike. If we had followed the 10 basics listed below, we wouldn't have had to rely on luck.

10 Basics for Staying Safe on Your Hike

The following basics are for day hiking and for backpacking safety.

1. Have a plan.
2. Inform someone where you're going, and when you plan to return.
3. Keep a flashlight and whistle with you.
4. Eat well; stay hydrated: carry plenty of water.

5. Stay on the trail.
6. Ask for help when you need it!
7. Familiarize yourself with the area, and use an up-to-date map.
8. Expect changes in the weather; carry extra clothing and otherwise plan accordingly.
9. Take a basic medical kit with you.
10. Take a device for contacting the populated world.

Have a plan

For a day hike, your planning can be brief. You can get up in the morning and if you have the day free, find a hike in your favorite local hiking book or find a trail online. You can study a map of your city. In either case check distance, elevation gain, and trail difficulty. Bring a current map. Pack a bag, and with some driving, you can be on your way.

Inform someone of your hike

This may seem obvious, but it doesn't always happen. I live alone and go out for solo hikes often, so I make it a habit to let someone know when and where I'm going. Also let your contact know when you get back. Agree beforehand when your contact should alert rescue services if you haven't returned as planned.

Keep a flashlight and whistle with you

These are basic hiking equipment. The flashlight serves as a safety device in several ways: it can help you find your way in the dark (if for some reason you end up being out after dark), you can use it to startle and scare away unwanted wildlife, and it can serve as a locator device in case rescue workers are trying to find you. Get a flashlight with multiple light settings. You can wave it on high beam or use the blinking mode to draw attention if you're in a situation where you need to be rescued. Make sure you check your flashlight batteries before you take off, and/or carry extra batteries, depending on the length of your hike.

As for whistles, test yours on the trail with your hiking partner. You can't hear all whistles in the woods or in canyons. Many whistles have the added usefulness of a built-in compass.

Eat and drink enough

When you hike, overeating is not usually a problem. Rather, be careful that you eat and drink enough. In Chapter 13 I wrote to always carry a snack and emergency food when you go out into any wilderness. With a sudden weather change, you can remedy and prevent dehydration or hypothermia by adequate water and food intake.

Stay on the trail.

One day I was hiking alone in a natural park in the San Francisco Bay Area. Marked trails crisscrossed the park, so I didn't see the need for a compass.

I had a simple tourist map that showed where the trails were. I had agreed with my family when I would return. I had taken care of basic safety by telling someone approximately where I would hike (I hadn't told them which trail in the park I would follow); I had water and food, and I had a map. Despite these precautions, at one point the trail markers confused me and I took a wrong turn.

I realized I'd been hiking away from my point of return when I saw far below me the roof of a school I knew was several miles from my exit point. I had to change directions to get back to my car. I found a trail with a private property sign on it but walked around the gate, and based on the sun's position in the sky, followed it in the direction I figured I needed to go. It was a hot, sunny day. I was sweating and had only one water bottle with me.

I felt some anxiety about making it back on time, but I didn't panic. It took more than an hour to get to a point I recognized. I'd hiked through gullies and around canyons, never knowing if the next ridge was the one that could lead to my car. For a while, there was no cell phone reception so I couldn't call my family.

Finally I was able to alert them that I would return later than we had agreed. Stopping often to assess my location, I finally got myself out of the network of trails in which I'd been lost.

This anecdote shows how easy it is to get into trouble if unprepared, even on a day hike close to civilization. If I had slipped, or twisted or broken an ankle in my hurry to get back, I could have been stuck in a canyon, run out of water, been without cell phone reception, and waiting hours for someone to find me, since my family doesn't worry quickly.

I was prepared for some emergencies, but not for getting lost. I had not carried my SPOT (my emergency GPS device); I had not brought enough water. I had my whistle, but I had no light or fire starter, which would have been dangerous to use in the flammable California canyons. What saved me from real trouble was my ability to stay calm, to orient myself in the terrain, and to hike farther than planned.

Ask for help.

Don't be shy about asking another hiker if you're on the right trail when you're hiking alone. Ask other hikers where they're coming from or where they're going, and tell them where you want to go. Exchanging information among hikers is of lifesaving value, as the first story in this chapter shows. Not only can another hiker redirect you if you are going the wrong way, but another person knowing you're out hiking, and maybe knowing your name, can mean the difference between being found and not being found. In the Himalayas (and I'm sure in the Andes and other high mountain regions), people habitually greet each other and talk on the trail. This isn't just a friendly, cultural behavior; greeting each other is part of surviving in the high mountains. It can be lifesaving when you leave your urban detachment at home.

Familiarize yourself with the area and carry a map.

A map is your guide for staying on the trail or leading you back to it. It is foolhardy to go on a hike without a hard-copy map. Even though you may use your smartphone or GPS, batteries are not reliable and electrical charges are sometimes scarce. A map and compass are necessary guides for finding your way out of the wilderness when you have to leave the familiar trail; if the weather turns, or if you experience physical problems, you may need to find a shortcut back to the trailhead or to a road where you can be picked up. A map will show you side trails to the populated world in case you need them.

Take a basic medical kit with you.

You can use a ready-to-go mountaineering first-aid kit or make your own. I prefer to make my own and adapt my first-aid kit to the circumstances of my hike. In the backpacking section of this book, I describe the medical kit that needs to contain bandages, some sterile gauze, alcohol wipes, and a bandage for wrapping gashes. With the spread of ticks carrying Lyme disease I have added a tick-removing tool and a little box to carry the tick out for testing.

Take a device for contacting the populated world.

Asking for help when you need it works best if you have a device that allows you to contact the populated world. This device can begin with a cell phone. If your hike takes you out of cell phone range, a GPS device will keep you connected to the populated world. I use a GPS safety device called a SPOT, for my hiking adventures. A SPOT differs from a GPS mapping device in that when I push the SOS button, the SPOT will broadcast my location and set a rescue mission in motion. It's money well spent. The yearly subscription and initial cost of the device is reasonable. There are several rescue devices on the market with different features, such as InReach, a device that allows you to send text messages via satellite. The devices made for the army have the surest data transmission in case of an accident, but they lack the feature of daily location broadcast and message capabilities. The SPOT sometimes has trouble contacting the satellite in forested terrain. I always look for an area open to the sky to send my transmissions and have had no trouble. Make your choice based on the hiking you'll be doing and where you will be.

Maps, GPS, Trail Profiles

You can get to know your trail before you set foot on it by reading and looking at pictures and available videos. The more you know about the area where you're going, the better your decisions on the trail can be and the safer you will be on your hike.

You can learn a lot more by reading maps of the area you in which intend to hike. Topographical maps (topo maps, for short) are available at outdoor stores, from forestry agencies, and online, either for sale or free to download. You can download GPS maps from the Internet to a GPS device or to an app on your phone.

Since I've been doing most of my long-distance hiking on the PCT and can use an app on my smartphone, I do not use a separate GPS device to guide me on the trail. But don't rely on the smartphone's app alone; it's important to have a back-up plan. Batteries can die on the trail. *Always* carry a hard-copy map!

Going on a hike in nature takes you away from people and easy access to help when you need it. For any outdoor adventure, I recommend bringing the basics, even if you're just going a mile away from "civilization."

Always carry water, food, a warm layer of clothing, rain protection, a basic medical kit, a survival blanket, a whistle, and a device to get in touch with civilization in case of emergency. Carrying the extra weight is well worth the peace of mind for you and your friends or family back at home.

The dangers I've pointed out are no reason to avoid hiking. Do you stay home because driving can be dangerous? Of course not, but you make sure you're able to drive safely. Hiking doesn't have to be a dangerous adventure if you use trail guides and bring the basic survival items.

Being prepared allows you to enjoy the surprises and beauty of the trail.

Trail Musings

It's the light that pulls me as it streams through my kitchen window in a late-summer yellow slant. Through the open window I can hear the crackle of the first leaves announcing fall. Inside there is the work that always waits to be done: the floor with its dusty crumbs, dishes in the sink, business tasks on the computer. But sensing the change in the air, the hint of autumn, I want to hold the warmth, light, and smells of summer just a little longer. I want to store the images and the smells in my brain for a long winter to come.

It's an easy decision, a quick look in the hiking book for a suitable trail to expand my lungs, stretch my legs, and move my arms with the swing of hiking poles for a day in nature instead of whirling around the kitchen with a mop in hand. Inside chores can wait. I'm going.

I add food, water, and a light jacket to my day pack, which already holds the basic hiking essentials such as a medical kit, a rain poncho, a whistle, a flashlight and my GPS device. I grab my sunhat, sun shirt, and hiking poles and am ready to hit the trail for the day. Remembering my new safety strategy, I quickly send a text to a friend, letting her know what I'm doing and when I expect to be back. Always one to sport a sense of humor, she texts back that she'll send a few strapping rescue guys out at 8:00 p.m. to come get me and bring along the beer. In the excitement of giving myself a day off, I almost forget to take my camera. A journal for writing gets added. I can already see a grassy spot near a lake for putting thoughts on paper.

A 45-minute drive puts me at the trailhead. I see only one other car: I may have the trail to myself today. Slight anxiety about being out alone mixes with confidence about knowing how to find my way, and is soon absorbed by the familiar rhythm of moving my arms and legs at 2 mph, my breathing sped up as the trail gently climbs. Where will this tunnel of conifers take me today? Deep green of the trees is all around, rising tall to the sky. Flowers and grasses of summer have dried into a brown carpet where the fungi wait for fall rains. The route loops around a dried-up lake, bits of marshy green and brown mud, too dry for mosquitoes.

I'm glad I chose this trail today, so often inaccessible because of the swarms of mosquitoes in summer. The sun is high, sending dazzling light through the trees, soft light that seems to brush the skin of my arms. Sunlight stored in my brain is a source of happiness. Can happiness be stored? I wonder.

After about 6 miles, as my stomach rumbles, I come around another bend and there lies a rippling, shimmering teal-colored lake, large enough to invite me for a swim. A bunch of boulders, warm and smooth to the touch, offer a seat near the water's edge. Ignoring my stomach, I strip for this late-summer silky bath. I jump, shiver as I feel the cold depth below and swim to acclimate. Soon I drift, body stretched out on the warm surface water, held in nature's embrace. I may be a woman without a partner, but I'm sure not feeling alone right now. The world of water, sun, and light is my friend and comfort. After a while I emerge from my water musings and climb ashore to fill my rumbling stomach. The joy of prickling skin as the breeze dries me against a warm boulder and the satisfaction of a hearty sandwich fully meet my needs at the moment.

A soft whirring draws my attention to the water's edge. Two dragonflies circle each other until they connect, mating in flight with a blue dazzle of wings. I have no one to do this dance with. Do I miss it? Not now, not here. I'm filled with love of light, fresh smell of pine, and sharp-tinged dry grasses. I'm fulfilled, I'm whole.

Another 6 miles, my body soon moves along the rocky trail. By the end of the day, the bottoms of my feet are warm and massaged, my limbs slack with a satisfied fatigue, and my mind and heart are humming with happiness from a day well spent. I don't need to be rescued, and I don't need a beer to wind down at the end of day.

Section III

BACKPACKING

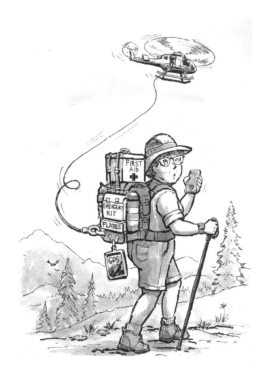

Trail Musings

The path in front of me stretches into a tunnel of green trees. Cold morning air swishes through like a message from another place. I am southbound for 300 miles. The tunnel is a long out-breath dismissing everyday life, the responsible life, my life that has been lacking the big spark.

I take my first steps loaded with water, food, and survival gear. I'm off on an adventure to find that spark again. The tree tunnel chills my excitement and drops me into the movement of arms and legs. The roots and rocks on the path draw my attention further to my feet. I'm walking, breathing, finding my rhythm, a rhythm that will become the music of living on the trail.

I'm clean at this point. I don't fit into these woods. A northbound hiker comes speeding in my direction, with dusty, tattered running shoes, dusty beige shorts, no shirt, unkempt hair flying, dirty hands moving his hiking poles like paddles in a river, water bottle bouncing off his pack. A breathless hello. "How far is Timberline Lodge? I'm hungry for a big breakfast," he says. He's the first of many hikers who'll come from the south in the weeks to come, from a mysterious faraway land beyond snowy mountain passes, hot lava fields, desert, and deep woods.

Many of them have stepped out of ordinary life to live four or five months on the trail. Many of them will meet themselves in new ways as their bodies and minds are doing the dance of simplicity and daily discipline.

I'm fresh on the trail, and my gray shirt is shiny. My pants are a pristine green. My pack is silvery with a bright orange top. My mind is eager, my body plump.

The tunnel is sucking me in. There's a window in the green walls of trees opening on a photo moment of Mount Hood. I stand and plant a little seed of thought about a climb to its snowy peak. Five years ago I did such a climb. Five years and a lifetime of experiences ago. Five years and loss of love. The big spark that sustained my everyday living has gone out. I'm here to find that spark again. I turn to the path and start walking.

15: Where the Path Will Take YOU

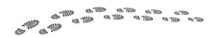

Planning is dreaming. What better thing to do on a stormy winter night sitting by the fire than read about places to go?

When you're ready for backpacking, follow the same pattern as for a day hike: nurture the idea, look at your destination options, choose one, and create a plan. For a multiday trip, the planning becomes more complex and a vital part of your journey.

Planning a multiday hike happens before you train, before you get your gear, before you're ready to leave home. Planning is dreaming. What better thing to do on a stormy winter night while sitting by a fire than read about places you want to visit? Start by collecting hiking magazines or hiking books, and scroll through hiking websites and social media to find scenic trails nearby a few months ahead of the day you want to start your trip.

To avoid pressure and to lower anxiety caused by the many details involved in a long trip, start your preparations several seasons in advance. The longer you've decided to stay on the trail, the farther ahead you must plan, prepare gear and food, and train your body. Once you've done a long trip, the outfitting phase will be shorter, but gathering food and training will take just as long as for your first long trip.

Divide your planning into several stages to make it a pleasure rather than a chore.

1. Dreaming. Let yourself fantasize, gather information, talk to people about hikes they have taken, look at pictures, browse through guidebooks, watch videos, or join a Facebook hiking group where you can hear about and see photos of places you never dreamed of. Bookmark interesting hikes and organize them into a file on your computer, or put sticky notes on pages if you have a printed guidebook. This is fun and helps you get into the spirit of walking and hiking.

2. Narrowing your options. Get real about your schedule, your finances, your other responsibilities, and whether you want to hike with friends or go alone, and pick a few trips that might be possibilities. Talk to others whom you might want as company on your trip. This will reveal how serious you are about taking the big hike. If you want to do this, you'll hear a voice inside you whisper, "GO!" I always ask myself, "Am I ready to go out alone if no one wants to join me?" And if I do the hike by myself, "What trip am I willing to do alone?" That way, I don't have to feel let down or desperate if no one comes out of the woodwork to hike with me.

Of the five people who show interest, usually only one will make the commitment and see it through. Remember you were the dreamer; the others have to come on board and give into the spirit of the trail.

3. Getting down to the details. Read guidebooks about the possible trips you have chosen. How far away do you have to drive to get to the trail? How accessible is the trail? How do you get to the trailhead? Is there a bus you can take to get there, or do you need to depend on others for a ride? For longer trips, this becomes a point of decision making, since you might not want to leave your car at one end of the trail, only to have to go back and get it weeks or months later.

Who can drop you off? Who will do so? What hiking support system will you use for food resupplies, drop-offs, and bailouts (this applies to the longer hikes)? For multiday hikes, you can usually leave your car at the trailhead, hike out and return the same way, or do a loop. If you have a hiking partner, you can opt to put a car at both ends of the trail you're going to hike, which takes care of your transportation to the trail and back. A third option is a shuttle service that will move your car from the trailhead to the end of the trail. If you're poised between doing a multiday hike and a longer hike, don't fret about the decision, because a few multiday training hikes are necessary anyway before tackling a longer trek for training purposes. Ease of access and vicinity will be more important deciding points than beauty and locale in this case. If you can get both, lucky you.

4. Narrow down the date(s). These will depend on your availability, your hiking partner's, and the best time to hike the trail. Once you decide, you can begin the work of scheduling.

5. Trip specifics. Read guidebooks, blogs, and get on a Listserv connected to the hike of your choice to learn about its features—glories and quirks. Remember you are most likely not the first to hike this trail, so learn from others' experiences. You will compile a list of needed gear, food, a water purification system, and footwear. You will check the gear you have and acquire what you need. If you give yourself enough planning time, you can look for sales and find discount gear items.

6. Tying the knot. You're now ready to commit. You arrange your transportation to the starting point of your hike, make your lodging arrangements near that starting point; tet a firm commitment from your support person for pickup at the end, food drops, and emergency pickup; and pin down public transportation schedules to and from the trail. Don't let the lack of a support person stop you from going on a long hike. Plenty of people access on their own the trailheads of the Pacific Crest Trail (PCT), Appalachian Trail (AT), and Continental Divide Trail (CDT), the three big long-distance hiking trails in North America. They use public transportation, hitch-hike or avail themselves of local "trail angels" all the time. Then again, if you have friends or family living near your trail starting point, it makes it easier to get on the trail.

7. Organize, train, pack. Here's the last and final stage of preparation.

- Plan your training or continue with training you've started.
- Create a gear list and get the items you've decided you need for your chosen trip. Beside the gear list in the appendix, you can get gear lists online or in the back of guidebooks. You can look at gear lists on YouTube, where an avid hiker will lay it all out for you.
- Create a hiking schedule. For long trips you can plan your day-to-day itinerary, figuring out how many miles

you will cover each day and where and when your food resupply stops will be. You can create a hiking schedule based on elevations, mileage, difficulty of terrain, and needed rest days, called zero days in trail vernacular to indicate 0 miles hiked. This way you can figure out how much food you will need and how much food you must carry between resupply stops. Since these daily hiking plans are notorious for not working out, you can leave your daily schedule up to chance and let your body, mood, and the weather dictate how far you'll hike. You can find food supplies along the way, or you can send yourself supplies a few stops ahead.

Training

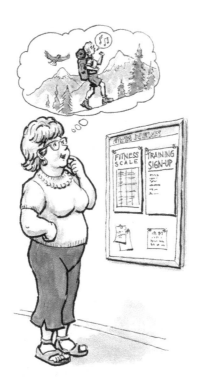

16: Getting Ready for the Distance

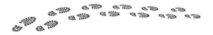

The best physical exercise to get in shape for hiking is walking. Walking is slow, methodical, repetitive, and low-impact, and anyone can do it. It's also the main component of hiking.

Already being a walker, I didn't just pack my bag and start hiking the Pacific Crest Trail (PCT). Some people do. You can read the wry, funny, and not-so-funny stories of Bill Bryson walking the Appalachian Trail and Cheryl Strayed walking the PCT that illustrate what can happen if you load up your pack and start without training.

Recently I met some people on the first part of the PCT who were dressed in sweatshirts and long pants, carrying a pack that looked like it weighed at least 40 pounds. They were standing by the side of the trail, catching their breath. They asked me if the trail would get steeper. I told them this incline was nothing compared with the Sierras. I encouraged them to think in terms of 1 mile at a time, reminding them they had already walked 20. I didn't think they would make it.

I met them again in a resupply town; they told me they had ditched a lot of their load, gone home to rethink what they were doing, and were building their training into their day on the trail, slowly increasing their daily mileage. If you're young, maybe you'll survive it, but if you're over 50, you invite injury and a divorce from Mother Nature.

It can start with a thought, a thought that excites you, that lets you dream beyond the ordinary, that inspires an emotional bounce, gives you hope for a better life. You feel yourself rise to a challenge. Instead of letting your age shrink you, you let your accumulated years be a force of expansion and turn you into a more alive person.

You don't have to take on the 2650-mile PCT challenge to find more vitality. You may take on a 3-day backpack challenge and see what it's like. You may take on a 50-mile challenge and find out how it changes you. Life is change. It's up to you to guide the change in a positive or negative direction, to take whatever has come your way and let it push the edges of your status quo, loosen its constraints.

Who can say, "My life is perfect as it is"? Your life may be good, and maybe you're content, but that doesn't mean there isn't room to expand the positives now and in the future. Here's what it takes to do this via *backpacking*.

Chapter 10 described what it takes to walk or hike 5 miles. The following chapters outline training schedules for 5–50-mile backpacking trips and 50–500-mile long-distance hikes! Training charts are also available in the appendix.

To walk day after day, you must be strong and have a well-functioning body. As we age, our walking posture and our strength change, partially because of sarcopenia, loss of skeletal muscle and resulting loss of function. Inactive people can lose as much as 3 to 5 percent of their muscle mass per decade after age 30.

According to Mary Lowth, MD, "Age-related changes in the balance of older persons result in compensatory responses that meet routine needs but may be ineffective under demanding circumstances." The American College of Sports Medicine (ACSM) recommends that "able-bodied adults" do strength training 2 to 3 times a week for at least 20 to 30 minutes. For women (and men) over 50, strength training is important to support balance, prevent falls, prevent or reduce osteoporosis, reduce back problems, and help maintain muscle mass.

Even though walking strengthens your body, specific strength training is important if you intend to carry a pack for any distance. Thus base strength is important to develop in the months leading up to a longer hiking adventure. Sufficient base strength to carry a pack over long distances is not something you can build in 6 weeks.

If you can't walk a mile without pain today, you may have to create a 3-year plan for yourself to walk 500 miles carrying a pack. It's possible, but it won't happen quickly. If you exercise consistently and can hike 5 miles without negative side effects, you can train and be ready for a longer hike in 6 months. To find out where you are on the fitness scale, speak to the trainer in your gym if you have one, or do one or more of the standard available fitness tests available on the internet, such as a step test for aerobic fitness, a balance test, and a muscular strength test. You can find links to sample tests in the appendix. Knowing your fitness level helps you decide what training you need. To improve your strength, do strength-training exercises at least twice a week.

Good body structure means you have a body that can walk without ill effect. It means that your legs, your back, and your hips are in working order and in decent alignment. If you have alignment problems, consult with a physical therapist (or someone who can rework connective tissue) and with a chiropractor to help correct spinal alignment. Small alignment problems can become big problems once you're on the trail carrying a pack.

A Warning!

Before you embark on walking distances make sure you speak with your physician and get the go-ahead to begin your training. If you have undetected health problems, you might find that the stress of training exacerbates your problem and sets you up for injury. You need your heart, lungs, and organs in working order to enjoy this ambitious aspect of the walking life.

17: From 5 to 50 Miles in 8 Weeks

Trail Musings

> I am answering the call: "Step out, walk away from phones, Wi-Fi, and people. Find the empty place, discover yourself anew." My feet in their comfortable walking shoes are my aides, as are my legs, held together by the scar tissue and re-grown tendons of age and injury. My back, leaning into the light netting of the pack frame, is my genetic code, strong and flexible. My will, coached by my father's tenacity, supported by my mother's hand, is my fuel source.

If you've become a walker, a time may come when you're ready for more than a 5-mile walk or just another day hike. Spring may be around the corner and you are dreaming of trips into nature for the summer. Or the heat of summer is over, and cooler fall days are inviting you out again. Maybe you want to escape winter in the Northern Hemisphere and hike in New

Zealand, or go to Machu Picchu to explore high elevations. In the United States, we have miles and miles of developed nature trails available. Unlike Europe, the Himalayas, and parts of South America, the United States trails are not dotted with towns and villages accessible for an overnight stay. Thus when you go out into nature for any length of time, you have to carry everything you need in a backpack or bring pack animals. If you can walk 5 miles comfortably and have developed your core (torso) and leg strength, you can put on a backpack, load it with your gear, hope it isn't too heavy, and go for an overnight hike into the mountains, hiking 5–7 miles each day. It's a good start.

If you want to do a 50-mile backpack trip, which will take 4 to 6 days, you must train. You will need to be a regular walker/hiker, with interval training and weight training in your schedule. Two or three months before you plan to go out, adopt a training schedule to get yourself ready. While you're training for your vacation, you'll be getting a taste of what's ahead. At the same time you'll be expanding your get-away options for the future.

The 8-Week Training Schedule

An 8-week training format follows these principles,

1. Make walking a daily part of your life
2. Do a cross-training routine twice a week. (See options below.)
3. Increase the distance weekly
4. Start on flat terrain
5. Increase elevation gain weekly, with more elevation gain over a certain distance, thereby increasing the incline
6. Carry a weighted pack

7.   Increase the pack weight weekly

By the end of 6 to 8 weeks, you'll be able to walk/hike between 3 and 6 times your initial distance. (The longer the distance you start with, the less your distance will increase, because your body has its natural limits.) You'll hike with 3 to 6 times the weight you started with (the more weight you start out with, the smaller the increase in weight will be), and you'll increase elevation gain by 3 to 6 times your initial elevation gain (again, elevation gains will be less if the initial inclines are greater). The following schedule is only a guideline; you can make adjustments as your circumstances dictate.

This is how your weekly schedule may look.

5 TO 50 MILES TRAINING SCHEDULE							
	MON	TUE	WED	THURS	FRI	SAT	SUN
WEEK 1	Rest	Cross-training 45 min.	Walk-hike 3 miles	Weight training 30 min.	Cross-training 45 min.	Hike 5 miles	Walk-hike 3 miles
WEEK 2	Rest	Cross-training 45 min.	Walk-hike 3.5 miles	Weight training 30 min.	Cross-training 45 min.	Hike 6 miles	Walk-hike 3.5 miles
WK 3	Rest	Cross-training 1 hour	Hike 4 miles, 500 ft. elevation gain	Weight training 40 min.	Cross-training 1 hour	Hike 7 miles, 500 ft. elevation gain	Walk-hike 3 miles, 500 ft. elevation gain
WEEK 4	Rest	Cross-training 1 hour	Hike 4 miles, 500 ft elevation gain	Weight training 40 min.	Cross-training 1 hour	Hike 7 miles, 750 ft. elevation gain	Weight training 40 min.
WEEK 5	Rest	Cross-training 1 hour	Hike 4 miles, 500 ft. elevation gain	Weight training 40 min.	Cross-training 1 hour	Hike 8 miles, 1000 ft. elevation gain, carry 10 lbs.	Hike 3 miles, 500 ft. elevation gain, carry 10 lbs.

5 TO 50 MILES TRAINING SCHEDULE							
WEEK 6	Rest	Cross-training 1 hour	Hike 3 miles, 500 ft. elevation gain, carry 15 lbs.	Weight training 40 min.	Cross-training 1 hour	Hike 9 miles, 1250 ft. elevation gain, carry 15 lbs.	Hike 4 miles, 500ft. elevation gain, carry 15 lbs.
WEEK 7	Rest	Weight training 1 hour	Hike 3 miles, 500 ft. elevation gain, carry 15 lbs.	Weight training 40 min.	Cross-training 1 hour	Hike 10 miles, 1500 ft. elevation gain, carry 20 lbs.	Hike 4 miles, 500 ft. elevation gain, carry 20 lbs.
WEEK 8	Rest	Cross-training 1 hour	Hike 3 miles, 500 ft. elevation gain, carry 20 lbs.	Weight training 40 min.	Cross-training 1 hour	Hike 12 miles, 2000 ft. elevation gain, carry 20 lbs.	Hike 4 miles, 500 ft. elevation gain, carry 20 lbs.

Notice that I've set two consecutive hiking days to get your body used to hiking and carrying multiple days in a row. Also I scheduled the longer time consuming hikes on the weekend, assuming that's when people who work have their free time. Of course you can move training days to fit your work schedule.

If you're short on time and feel strong enough, you can condense this training schedule to 6 weeks. But you might be more sore as you increase your distances and weight faster. If you plan a longer hike on level terrain, you can drop the increased incline in weeks 7 and 8.

Cross-training can take the form of any aerobic, muscle-developing exercise: bicycling, dancing, rowing, playing tennis, playing racquetball, roller-skating, cross-country skiing, or any activity that makes you happy and keeps you interested in moving. Yoga is a wonderful antidote for sore muscles and creates flexibility, but it doesn't build much strength unless you do power yoga. Strength and endurance are the goals of your training for the 50-mile distance. Your flexibility will increase the more you walk/hike. If you have time, do a few (yoga) stretches after a hike or at the end of a busy workday, to create calm and relaxation and keep your muscles from tightening.

You can take a strength-training class for 50-plussers at your gym, or work with a trainer, especially if you have never performed a strength routine. You may follow a routine at home that involves lifting weights, and doing push-ups, planks, curls, squats, lunges, pull-ups and tricep dips if you are familiar with these exercises. The muscles you need on the trail are biceps and triceps for lifting and carrying, core muscles for carrying, strong quads and hamstrings for climbing and descending. You will create strong flexible feet by doing exercises standing on your toes with your feet arched (squats, knee flexes with a ball, and more).

Summarized like this, the suggested training may overwhelm you. Remember, you can enter this world of walking by expanding it gradually. You can add routines one at a time, and the body will remember and be grateful for each expansion. Training will begin to feel like living. Let the joy you feel after a hike, or a workout, be the barometer for your training schedule.

18: A Woman at Her Own Speed

On my sixth day of hiking the John Muir trail in the Sierra Nevada, I met a Japanese woman. She looked likely to be past 50 years of age. Her skin was creased, her hair gray. She wore a blue shirt and had a colored handkerchief in her hand and one around her neck. She was alone. Resting her pack against a rock, she wiped her brow.

I stopped and asked, "How far are you hiking?"

She answered, "I'm hiking the whole JMT."

"Are you hiking solo?" I asked.

"Yes, I hike by myself."

"How many miles are you doing a day?" The woman appeared older than me, and I was curious what her hiking pace was.

"I go slow, I rest when I need to, but I get there. Don't know what my average daily mileage is, but I have been on the trail for 2 weeks," she answered.

I did a quick calculation in my head. We were 90 miles from the start of the trail. With a rest day, it meant she was hiking maybe 7 miles a day, going over a high pass almost daily.

"How old are you, if I may ask?" I hadn't met many people older than myself on the trail, so I wondered.

"I'll tell you, if you promise not to tell. They'll send me home if they know my age. I am 70 years old. I didn't tell my children. They will come get me." She snickered. "I wanted to do this. I don't want others to stop me."

"Are you having a good time?" I asked.

"Very good. I meet people from Japan and talk with them. Walking is in my blood."

I had met several Japanese people hiking this trail. One man had told me he was doing the 220 miles for the fourth time. Images from stories of sturdy Japanese people making pilgrimages into the mountains flashed in my brain. I believed her. She would do this putting one foot in front of the other.

I thought about this woman as I hiked on with my party. She was doing what she wanted. It wasn't about challenging herself; she hiked the trail because a thought had gotten hold of her. She had told no one. She had left her home for a vacation, and would tell about her adventure only when she returned. Was what she was doing safe? Considering how many people were on the trail, she would probably be okay if something happened. I hiked on, eager to reach our resupply point that night.

Two days later at John Muir Ranch where we had rested and resupplied, the Japanese woman walked in with a smile. She was moving at her own speed. She was having her experience of delight.

19: From 50 to 500 Miles in 3 Months

Trail Musings

> *I want the experience. The experience of oozing in my skin when sunlight warms me after a cold dawn. The experience of heaviness in my limbs when dogged walking propels me beyond what my mind thinks my body can do. The experience of edgy alertness as I traverse a narrow ledge. I want to experience my aloneness in the vastness of nature, the smallness of my being under the starry sky. I want to love myself while in the experience. I want the experience to tell me who I am.*

Hiking 50-plus miles will show you who you are. They require not only more time to complete, but more training. Just as you have to maintain a fitness base for the 50-mile distance, for the 100- to 500-mile distance, your training needs to be ongoing to support a level of fitness you can crank up a few months before you go out on your long hike. For the longer hikes, you don't need to be *more* fit than for the 50-mile hikes, but a 50-plus woman (or man) must realize that the body is less forgiving when it comes to mistakes in hiking and training. When you overexert yourself, you don't bounce back as you did in younger years. When you exert yourself day in, day out on the trail without proper training, you may injure yourself and regret you ever got started.

One 50-year-old man I met on the trail had a successful tech-company career. He decided he needed to get away from his stressful life to reorient himself. Used to a moderate workout schedule 3 times a week, he considered himself athletic and strong. He figured that with a few weeks of stepping it up, he could embark on the John Muir Trail and hike the 220 miles as long as he kept an easy pace.

I encountered him a day past Donahue Pass at 10,000 feet of elevation amid a drenching rain that hadn't dampened his enthusiasm. I met him again past John Muir Ranch. Having developed pain in his lower leg, he had taken a few days off to let his calf recover. He figured with rest the pain would go away.

It didn't. The 2 weeks of pushing himself had created a stress injury that took 2 months to heal. He had no choice but to hike (hobble?) out from the trail earlier than planned.

When he contacted me later, I learned he'd been on crutches for 6 weeks to let his leg heal. Two years later he hadn't gone back to the trail. He had realized that he wasn't young any longer, that he couldn't just get up and go as he always had. The experience was an eye-opener for someone successful in the larger world, someone who didn't think in terms of decline.

The injuries of distance hiking are stress injuries, a knee that becomes unhappy from climbing and descending, a hamstring insertion that tears and whines every time you take a step, feet that ache because they can't hold up the weight, or a lower back that may spasm from straining because of the lack of core muscle. Has your body lifted weights, so you can hoist that pack day in, day out? Have you done your push-ups so you can push yourself uphill with your hiking poles without developing deltoid pain? On a short distance, this doesn't occur, but on the long distance your overall body fitness needs to be excellent to keep going.

The training schedule I've developed has been tested by my students, who can enjoy their 200-plus-mile hikes, have few body discomforts, and walk out of the wilderness without injury while talking about the next long hike they want to do. After age 50, too many weeks of training (I'm not saying too hard) are better than too few.

If you are reading this book, you already know that physical decline is unavoidable. For a healthy person who wants to walk long distances, the decline in tissue resilience is the greatest challenge.

After age 50, you can't afford to exercise intermittently, and stay in shape. After age 50, exercise and movement have to become part of your daily life if you want to feel good, stay healthy, and take on new adventures.

For the long distances, you will want to walk in your off-season while keeping up your strength-building exercises (yes, push-ups, pull-ups, planks, dead lifts, and so on). You'll want to include aerobic exercise which pushes you to use your muscles differently than for walking.

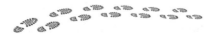

If you have body parts compromised from past accidents or injuries that can act up under duress, figure out special exercises to do. Talk to your physical therapist to get reha-bilitation exercises.

The 3-month training schedule for longer hikes is like the training schedule for the 50-mile hikes, except that the training lasts 3 months instead of 2 months, the cross-training has to be more serious, and you must add stretching to your weight training so your body can handle the increased weight training.

The basic components of the 3-month training routine are the same as for the 5–50-mile hike:

1. Walk/hike with an incline, increasing pack weight over time
2. Engage in some form of cross training
3. Do weight training and stretching

This training format will get you ready for the 100–500-mile stretches averaging 12-14 miles of hiking daily. If you want to decrease your daily distance on the trail, you can adjust the training schedule accordingly. For each of the 3 months of your training, you will set a weekly goal and increase distance, elevation, and weight, week by week. The greatest gain in strength and aerobic capacity will occur in the second month. The third month serves to maintain and solidify your fitness. Then taper off and rest before you go on your long hike.

It should speak for itself that if you want to hike at altitudes above 6000 feet, training at higher altitudes is helpful. If you cannot train at higher altitude because of where you live, climb stairs for upward-movement training. You will have to include time in your trip schedule for altitude adjustment in the initial days of your hike.

The 3-Month Training Schedule

Month 1: Ramp up your base.

Six days a week of training, one day of rest. A rest day should include movement, just not hauling rocks for your garden up an incline or mowing the back 40 acres with a hand mower. Aim for activities that demand little effort and little physical repetition, except maybe playing your piano or hitting the keyboard on your computer.

On training days, rotate walking/hiking one day, cross-training another, and strength building yet another. You can combine a hiking day with a stretching session afterward, or a cross-training session with a short strength-building routine. For bodies over 50, a minimum of 2 days off between sessions of strength training allows for the muscles to rebuild, yet more than a 4-day lag between sessions stops the process of building muscle.

In the first month, you can hike up to 8 miles, but 6 miles is enough. You need to carry only what you need on your hike, such as water, extra clothing, camera, and a snack. Your cross-training should comprise a steady, moderate workout. For different cross-training activities see Chapter 17.

For strength building do at least a 20-minute weight-training routine with different exercises, such as push-ups, pull-ups, stomach curls, planks, leg lifts, and squats. Start where you feel comfortable, and then increase the frequency, weight, and time of each exercise gradually. If you experience a mild soreness on interim days, you know the training is working.

50 TO 500 MILES TRAINING SCHEDULE MONTH 1							
	MON	TUES	WED	THURS	FRI	SAT	SUN
WEEK 1	rest from formal training	Cross-training 45 min.	Walk/hike 3 miles	Weight training 20 min. stretch 10 min.	Cross-training 45 min.	Hike 5 miles, stretch 5 min. after	Walk/hike 3 miles, stretch 5 min. after
WEEK 2	Rest	Cross-training 45 min.	Walk/hike 3.5 miles	Weight training 30 min. stretch 10 min.	Cross-training 45 min.	Hike 6 miles, stretch 10 min. after	Walk/hike 3.5 miles, stretch 5 min. after
WEEK 3	Rest	Cross-training 1 hour	Hike 4 miles, 500 ft. el-evation gain	Weight training 40 min. stretch 15 min.	Cross-training 1 hour	Hike 7 miles, 500 ft. el-evation gain, stretch 10 min. after	Walk/hike 3.5 miles, 500 ft. el-evation gain, stretch 10 min. after
WEEK 4	Rest	Cross-training 1 hour	Hike 4 miles, 500 ft. el-evation gain, stretch 5 min.	Weight training 40 min. stretch 15 min.	Cross-training 1 hour	Hike 7 miles, 750 ft. el-evation gain, stretch 10 min. after	Weight training 40 min., stretch 15 min. after

Month 2: Focus your efforts

This is the month to *maximize overall strength gain*. Your body can now work out daily with increasing intensity.

This is the month to *add weight* to your hiking, up to 15 pounds, and to increase elevation by 2000 feet. Your cross training should *include interval training*: this will improve your aerobic capacity.

This is also the month to *focus on your strength training*. Increase the number of your push-ups (20), modified pull-ups (15), crunches (30), plank time (60 seconds), squats (30x, and lifts up to 25 pounds.

Your mind may resist under all this pressure, and you'll feel tired and may want to quit. This resistance is usually more mental than physical. You're moving your fitness level up a notch. This second month trains you for the hard days on the trail when you need mental stamina to keep going.

Give yourself extra sleep time, and eat well (you will need more protein). Reward yourself once a week for following your training schedule. A massage does wonders after a rough week.

It may be cold or snowy if you start your training in late winter, making the idea of walking outside less pleasant. Actually it's an excellent setup for the emotional rewards you will get from the rigors of long-distance hiking.

50 TO 500 MILES TRAINING SCHEDULE MONTH 2							
	MON	TUES	WED	THURS	FRI	SAT	SUN
WEEK 5	rest from formal training	Cross-training 1 hour	Hike 4 miles, 500 ft. elevation gain, carry 10 lbs.	Weight training 40 min. stretch 15 min.	Cross-training, steady work-out 1 hour	Hike 8 miles, 1000 ft. elevation gain, carry 10 lbs., stretch 10 min.	Walk-hike 3 miles, 500 ft. elevation gain, stretch
WEEK 6	Rest	Cross-training 1 hour	Hike 3 miles, 500 ft. elevation gain, carry 15 lbs.	Weight training 40 min. stretch 15 min.	Cross-training, steady work-out 1 hour	Hike 8 miles, 1250 ft. elevation gain, carry 15 lbs., stretch	Hike 4 miles, 500 ft. elevation gain, carry 15 lbs., stretch

50 TO 500 MILES TRAINING SCHEDULE MONTH 2							
WEEK 7	Rest	Weight training 40 min., stretch 15 min.	Hike 3 miles, 500 ft. elevation gain, carry 15 lbs.	Weight training 40 min. stretch 15 min.	Cross-train-ing 1 hour	Hike 10 miles, 1500 ft. elevation gain, carry 20 lbs.	Hike 4 miles, 500-750 ft. eleva-tion gain, carry 20 lbs., stretch
WEEK 8	Rest	Cross-train-ing/ interval training 1 hour	Hike 3 miles, 500 ft. elevation gain, carry 20 lbs.	Weight training 40 min. stretch 15 min.	Cross-train-ing, steady work-1 hour	Hike 12 miles, 2000 ft. elevation gain, carry 20 lbs.	Hike 4 miles, 500-750 ft. eleva-tion gain, carry 20 lbs., stretch

Month 3: Peak and taper.

Pack weight: In the third month, if you live in or near moun-tainous terrain, you will hike with a full pack weight several times up a 2000-foot incline over a 4-mile stretch. If you live in flat terrain, you will have to use stairs or an elliptical trainer.

Elevation gains: Work up to the suggested elevation gains in the chart (1500-foot elevation gain over 5 miles to start).

Rest stops: When you are hiking with a full pack uphill, make sure you rest every hour for 10–15 minutes. For the long hikes it's helpful to adopt this routine. You should hike up to 12 miles at least by mid-month. Do this twice this month; then ease off for the next 2 weeks.

Overnight backpack trip: If you can fit another 3- or 4-day backpack trip in this month, do it. You'll really get your hiking legs under you that way. Then taper off from heavy hiking while you organize for the long trip to start 2 or 3 weeks later.

Cross training: In the third month keep up your cross-train-ing, while backing off from interval training to a moderate, pleasant workout.

Strength training: Do your strength training twice a week for the first 2 weeks, then taper to once a week while reducing the intensity of your workout.

	MON	TUES	WED	THURS	FRI	SAT	SUN
50 TO 500 MILES TRAINING SCHEDULE MONTH 3							
WEEK 9	Rest from formal training	Weight training 40 min., stretch 15 min.	Hike 4 miles, 500 ft. elevation gain, carry 20 lbs. stretch	Weight training 40 min. stretch 15 min.	Cross-training, steady workout 1 hour	Hike 12 miles, 1500 ft. elevation gain, carry 25 lbs., stretch	Hike 5 miles, 500 ft. elevation gain, carry 15 lbs., stretch
WEEK 10	Rest	Weight training 40 min., stretch 15 min.	Hike 5 miles, 500 ft. elevation gain, carry 20 lbs.	Weight training 40 min. stretch 15 min.	Cross-training, steady workout 1 hour	Hike 12 miles, 2000 ft. elevation gain, carry 25-30 lbs. stretch	Hike 5 miles, 500-750 ft. elevation gain, carry 20 lbs. ,stretch
WEEK 11	Rest	Cross-training, steady workout 1 hour	Hike 4 miles, 500 ft. elevation gain, carry 15 lbs. stretch	Weight training 30 min. stretch 15 min.	Cross-training, steady workout 1 hour	Hike 10 miles, 1500 ft. elevation gain, carry 25-30 lbs.	Hike 4 miles, 500 ft. elevation gain, carry 20lbs. stretch
WEEK 12	Rest	Cross-training, easy steady workout 45 min.	Hike 3 miles, 500 ft. elevation gain, carry 20 lbs.	Weight training 20 min. stretch 15 min.	Cross-training, easy steady workout 45 min.	Hike 8 miles, 1000 ft. elevation gain, carry 20 lbs.	Hike 3 miles, 500 ft. elevation gain, carry 15 lbs.

Maintain the same level of activity as in week 12 for the next few weeks. Rest the last week with normal daily activity. Your body is now ready to go on a long hike!

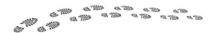

When you've achieved the daily discipline necessary for the trail, your mind will find freedom for thought and creativity.

Trail Musings

First light marks the forms of the world, long recognized as a time of awareness. First light lifts me out of a world of dreams where reality doesn't match what my conscious mind knows.

The bleeding sky, appearing as the light increases, gives back the world as I know it; is a reminder that there is more to living than meets the eye.

This knowing stays with me after I pack up my tent, hoist my pack, and start hiking. Bigger inside, straddled across different worlds, less fearful, I am aware that there is no place to go, no goal to reach.

Pressure on my shoulders from the weight of the backpack. Good pressure, squeezing me gently in the back. The pack wrapped around my hips embraces me, helps me lift my feet through my thighs with each step. Cool morning air brushes against my cheeks, stirs in my hair as the sun is sending soft rays through the trees. Each step matches the swing of my arms. My hands, placing the trekking poles a little ahead, pull me forward.

Step, swing, breathe, step, swing, breathe.

My eyes on the path in front of me, I scout for rocks, roots, and treads in the trail. I am moving my head with the swing of my step. A falling rock echoes the depth down below. Bird cry bounces against the steep wall rising above.

I walk in the center of the trail. The carved-out flat spot in front of me leads me to the next slope, the next pass, the next lake, the next valley.

These mountains are a big personality, a personality that requires my attention, my surrender.

This is what love is, complete absorption, complete contact, complete acceptance of what is given.

Through the trees, around the bend, on top of the pass, the vista erupts, sends shudders of pleasure through me. The landscape, larger than life, burns into my memory.

Outfitting

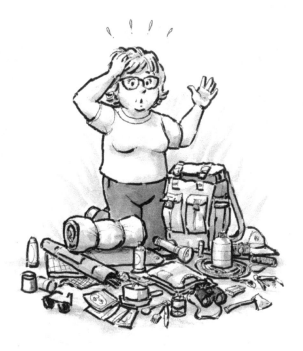

20: Gear for the Distance

When you hike longer distances, you won't just become intimate with nature, you will become intimate with your gear. The fit of your pack can support you or torture you. An extra loop on it can offer a place to hang a sweat rag within reach while you work your way up a cliff. A strap that rubs can make the difference between heaven and hell. Hiking means gear. Long-distance hiking means good gear. Remember the boot that rolled into the canyon in the movie *Wild*? That boot was an example of poorly chosen gear, causing blisters and pain. *Over long distances, gear matters, certain kinds of gear more than others.*

There is an abundance of gear available, which makes it difficult to wade through the options. *Backpacker* magazine is my trusted guide for this process. They publish a yearly issue foregrounding the best gear, a *Consumer Reports* version of the essential backpacking products: tents, sleeping bags, sleeping pads, backpacks, boots and shoes, and stoves. I am not getting paid to name them here, but the magazine will tell you what you need to know. Their staff tests a variety of products under a wide variety of conditions, then rates them for specific functions.

Is it important to get new gear? Not necessarily. You may already own useful items. Chances are, however, when you fill the pack you have with the gear in your possession, you will end up carrying more weight than is good for you.

Weight

When you are 50-plus years old, the less your pack weighs, the farther you'll be able to trek in a day and the less it will stress your precious body. Thus your joy in walking will increase. My advice for the average person over 50 is to keep your total pack weight under 30 pounds.

A practical way to calculate your pack weight is to calculate a percentage of your total body weight. The weight of your pack should only be 15–20 percent of your body weight. To get everything you need on the trail into a pack, including food and water, and keep it under 15–20 percent of your body weight, you have to choose lightweight gear.

Quality

As usual with purchases, quality counts. Lightweight gear can serve you only if it's high-quality gear, made of light materials that can stand up to use and abuse on the trail. There are no stores around the corner on the trail, and if your gear malfunctions, you will be left with primitive and temporary solutions. Choose your gear carefully; you will rely on it for your comfort and your safety.

Protection

Gear needs to protect you from the dangerous aspects of the elements: heat, cold, wetness, sun, and abrasion. Your shelter needs to keep you dry and warm. Your clothing needs to keep you warm or cool, depending on the temperatures, as well as dry and protected from sun and rain. Your footwear needs to protect you from rubs and bumps and support you for many miles.

Price

Evaluate each piece of gear for its weight, quality, and the protection it will give from the elements before you look at the price. If you compromise on any of these primary aspects, you put yourself at risk in the wilderness.

Midway in a 3-month training for a long summer hike, two trainees and I went out for an overnight in May in the woods of Oregon. It had been raining, and the forecast wasn't promising, but our schedules forced us into now-or-never mode. We figured it was a test hike, and we could always turn around if it became too wet. When we arrived at the trailhead, it wasn't raining. It was snowing! Optimism launched us onto the trail. We would get to test our rain gear!

Indeed the hiking kept us warm. By midday it had stopped raining and snowing, and there was a dusting of snow in the woods. We went on, shortening our route, and made camp in a spot we had chosen ahead of time. By 4:00 p.m. we had tents set up and were cozy, relaxing in our sleeping bags. We cooked our food in the vestibule of our tents, all the while making sure we stayed dry and warm. After dinner it rained again. I tied the extra tarp I had brought above my tent, which already had a rain fly, to give myself a bigger dry area outside my tent.

I fell into a long and deep sleep. When I awoke in the middle of the night to relieve myself, it was quiet. When I emerged from my tent, the light of my headlamp bounced back from a white ground. Snow, everywhere! It had been snowing and was snowing still, thus the quiet. I did my business and crawled back into my tent and sleeping bag, relishing the choice of my R-5 sleeping pad, made for sleeping on snow, and went back to sleep.

Morning presented a blue sky and full sun bouncing off a white landscape with a view of Mount McLoughlin covered in snow! The rope holding our food in a tree was frozen, and as I worked on getting the food bag down, my trainees emerged from their tents, tired and cold after a mostly sleepless night. They had been cold the whole time. Their sleeping bags were too thin and their sleeping pads inadequately insulated. Maybe I'm a warm sleeper and don't need as much insulation in the cold, but reasons aside, top-quality gear will pay off in comfort.

We ended up trudging through 5-foot snowdrifts, looking out at a picture-perfect white landscape to get back to the trailhead. It turned into a beautiful adventure, but if this had happened while on a longer hike, fatigue and weather exposure, wet boots, and thin sleeping bags would have become issues of safety.

When considering price, the price information *Backpacker* provides comes in handy. Their evaluation of gear takes price into account, helping you decide based on quality, protection, weight, *and* price. If you plan on hiking only in the summer, and know the weather well in your intended hiking areas, you can get away with a lighter, less expensive sleeping bag, and you might skip the tent and use a flimsy pad. This will work, *if* you can count on the temperatures. As you can see from my story, the weather may surprise you. On long hikes, you likely will go up to altitudes where the weather is unpredictable. If you are a 3-day or 4-day hiker, you can be less fussy over every ounce of weight, every bit of insulation, because you'll be carrying less food. If you want to go for longer hikes, you will *always* be grateful for better gear when foul weather hits.

I spent a summer in the Himalayas where the temperatures are around 80 degrees during the day and 50 degrees at night, even at high altitudes. It rarely rains in the summer, yet the summer I visited, the rains came, because of erratic monsoon weather patterns in the south. I got stuck in a rain/snowstorm for 3 days with wet gear. I learned that you can dry socks inside your sleeping bag with your body heat. My +10°F down sleeping bag did not get wet. My guide and horseman were less lucky. They slept under a tarp wrapped in wet blankets, huddled together to keep warm.

Over the last 10 years I have learned that light, high-quality gear is always worth it, and gradually I have been replacing my heavier gear, one or several pieces at a time. Outfitting from scratch for a long hike will run at least $1500 by 2017 prices. But top-quality gear will serve you for many years, so you can prorate the cost. Try staying in a hotel or B-and-B for a week; you'll spend as much and you won't have the uplifting experience of the outdoors.

21: Backpacking Gear Details

This book isn't intended to offer a complete guide for choosing your gear, but rather give a starting point for your research into the essential components of each piece of gear before you make your choices. Certain outdoor companies will let you test, use, and return your product if you don't like it or if it malfunctions, within a year of purchase. It's a great guarantee, one to watch for.

The Sleeping Bag

The sleeping bag is your shelter, your protection from low temperatures and hypothermia. Consider the following when choosing a sleeping bag:

Insulation: You must decide between down or polyester filling. Down is superior in its ability to keep you warm. When down gets wet, however, it's useless until it dries, and that can take a long time. Packing your down bag in a lightweight, waterproof, compression stuff sack (yes, all these features come in one product) can protect it from getting wet. If you sleep in a waterproof tent, your bag will be protected when it rains or snows at night.

Temperature rating: Err on the side of being too warm rather than too cold. Know your nighttime temperature needs by testing out a bag while sleeping in different nighttime temperatures. Take the 20°F, 30°F, etc. ratings with a grain of salt. Don't trust that your 20°F bag will keep you warm when temperatures dip to 20°F. You may be a cold or hot sleeper who needs more or less insulation to stay warm.

Weight and compactibility: Bags with poly filling can be light enough, but will be bulkier in a stuff sack than their equivalent in warmth in a down bag.

Price: Down bags are more expensive than polyester fiber bags.

The Sleeping Pad

The sleeping pad provides comfort, soothing your back for the next day of hauling weight. As we age, our bodies are less resilient and the effects of a day of walking on the trail stay with you longer than when you were younger. There are 2 types of sleeping pads.

Air-filled pads: If you can afford it, pamper yourself with an inflatable, lightweight, temperature reflective pad (it reflects your body heat, and provides insulation for sleeping on cold ground). Self-inflatable pads weigh more and don't offer as much cushioning as the blow-up pads.

Foam pads: The lightweight accordion-style foam pads are cheap and popular and might be worth a try before you invest more than a hundred dollars in a fancy inflatable pad. Many of the young hikers are comfortable with an accordion foam-style pad, but they have young, resilient bodies.

The Tent, Shelter

Your shelter protects you from the elements: sun, cold, rain, snow. When and where you plan to hike will determine whether you need a shelter. I have backpacked many 3-day and 4-day trips in the summer in southern Oregon without worrying about a shelter, beyond a light tarp for an occasional thunderstorm. Sleeping under the stars (cowboy camping) when mosquitoes and bugs aren't around is an uplifting experience.

For the places where it gets cold, and rainy, where the mosquitoes like it as much as you do, where snakes and scorpions crawl around at night, a shelter allows for a restful sleep. Consider the following features when choosing a shelter:

Weight: Because the tent is a big item in your sleep system, weight matters. Lightweight tents are expensive (in the $300 range). If you can, don't skimp on features.

Condensation: Shop for a tent with a low condensation rating; having condensation water dripping onto your bag and belongings makes for a miserable experience. Remember the need to keep a sleeping bag dry? Tents with a separate rain fly usually keep the inside tent dry, whereas single-layer tents build up condensation in damp, cold weather.

Freestanding versus staked: A freestanding tent looks great for those picture-perfect nights of camping on a rock plateau overlooking a canyon. At some point while camping out, the wind will come up and blow your tent around. Make sure you have a way to fasten your tent to the ground with tent pegs or to trees with guylines.

Tent versus hammock: I will do a pitch here for the back-packing hammock, my favorite go-to when I hike in forested terrain. The hammock allows the back to relax, and it elevates swollen legs for reverse blood flow after a long day of hiking. Mine allows me to sleep on my side wrapped in my cocoon with the stars visible through the mosquito netting above me. I let the rain fly dangle on the side. It has kept me dry in pouring rain.

The Backpack

Backpacker will feature best choices of the year in light-weight, comfortable packs. Few people use an external-frame pack anymore, but that doesn't mean your old and comfortable frame pack is a bad piece of equipment. When considering a new backpack, weigh these considerations:

External versus internal frame: The external frame holds the pack away from your back, allowing for airflow between your back and the load. Lightweight packs with external frames exist (made by Osprey) and, if fitted well, are a good choice.

Weight: The material of your pack can reduce your overall weight considerably. The new lightweight materials are strong even if the straps look narrow and the clasps are light. *Z-packs* and *UL* make ultra-light packs used by many thru-hikers. *Osprey* will replace your pack if something breaks, no questions asked. Even after five summers of hauling my rolling backpack around Europe, the company gave me a new one when a clasp closure ripped out during a flight.

Size: If you have a small pack, you won't be tempted to take too much stuff. A 45–55-liter size can hold all your backpacking needs for a longer trip and will certainly for a 4- to 5-day trip. If you backpack in winter and need more clothes and a warmer (which means heavier) sleeping bag, you'll need a larger backpack.

Comfort: When choosing a pack, pay attention to the comfort and ease of use of your hip belt and the comfort of the shoulder straps. Have an outdoor assistant help you fit the pack, or figure out what size you need. If you order online, you will need to have a friend measure you from C-7, the seventh cervical vertebra, to the iliac crest, the bony part of your pelvis in the back, to get an idea of size. This measurement will determine what size backpack you'll need. A size chart can convert your body measurement into pack size. Hip size can also determine your pack choice. When choosing a backpack check if the shoulder strap attachment is adjustable. The placement of the shoulder straps on the pack or frame determines the distribution of the pack weight on your back. The higher you carry the weight, the easier it is on your lower back.

Pack organization: Side, front, and top pockets are handy and allow for better organization of your contents. Certain lightweight packs are just one bag without outside pockets, which makes finding things more difficult. You could create inner pockets by using different-colored stuff sacks. However they add weight to the pack, and what you gain with getting a lighter, simple pack may be lost by adding the stuff sacks. A top pouch is a natural location for all the small items you want easy, quick access to on the trail, such as your medical kit.

Footwear

To boot or not to boot. You can tell a novice backpacker by her boots, they say. Heavy mountaineering boots are meant for just that, heavy mountaineering, such as Mount Everest. Most of the time heavy boots are unnecessary on the trail and add several pounds to every step you take. If you add that up for 8 hours of walking, you know what I mean.

When to use boots: I did a stretch of the PCT wearing my boots. Reports of difficult-to-cross snowfields and the need for micro-spikes, a traction device you can slip around the sole of your shoe/boot, made me choose more foot protection. After climbing for 6 hours over snow and big rocks off trail, the extra support and dry feet "outweighed" the advantage of a lighter hiking shoe. If you have weak ankles, aside from strengthening them on your walks/hikes, by all means give 'em the support of a boot when you are going out for longer, difficult hikes.

When to use shoes: For the long hikes on well-defined trails, a good hiking shoe will serve you. Cross-country running shoes are the choice of most younger hikers. I prefer a heavier hiking shoe with toe protection and good grip for crossing creeks and hiking on rocky trails. I started my long-distance hiking with Gore-Tex lined shoes. When the rain dripped into the shoes and my socks got wet, I sloshed for two days with wet feet. The boots and socks didn't dry until I let them dry out at home. Wet socks in shoes and boots are a recipe for blisters. There is a happy medium: the leather hiking shoe with breathable mesh, which allows your socks to dry out faster when they get wet. The shoe needs to be large enough to accommodate the swelling of your feet, which happens when you walk all day long. Blisters caused by tight shoes are a nuisance and can become debilitating.

Barefoot, minimal shoes: Many mountain people in the Himalayas and Andes go barefoot, tying their shoes to the load on their back. Their feet are strong, broad, and leathery. Living in a Western country, we aren't used to going barefoot on dirt and pavement. Even though there is a movement for minimal shoe-wear, I haven't seen people going minimal on the trail.

Socks: What you wear in your hiking shoe or boot is as important as the shoe. I recommend wool socks with or without a thin liner sock. They absorb sweat and keep your feet warm when it's cold even when the socks get wet. Some hikers in warmer climes prefer nylon socks that wash and dry quickly and can be changed frequently to avoid developing blisters. Whatever sock you choose, make sure you choose shoes large enough for your feet to expand. A half size larger than your normal shoe size is the recommendation for hiking shoes.

Hiking Poles

As I pointed out in Chapter 13, hiking poles can help you move. You don't have to be old and feeble to enjoy the benefits of your hiking poles. Poles help you move faster and steadier; they involve your arms and give your knees a break. For uphill stretches the poles help you pull yourself up; for the downhill, they work as brakes and support, taking the load off your knees. Poles are simple devices, and in a culture where we always try to sell something new, manufacturers have added a spring-loaded piece, and parts that extend, twist, and collapse for storage on some models. Here's a rundown on hiking poles:

Wooden sticks: Two sticks you find on the trail will do if you don't want to spend money on this piece of equipment.

Aluminum poles: Aluminum poles are light and strong enough for everyday use. They'll bend if they get stuck between rocks and you trip or move on. The length of the pole can be adjusted for different inclines.

Carbon fiber poles: Carbon fiber poles are the more expensive poles; they're stronger than aluminum ones and lighter. As with aluminum poles they extend and often collapse, and can have built-in suspension. I've not found the suspension significant enough to be worthwhile.

Collapsible versus noncollapsible poles: Collapsible poles have more parts and can therefore malfunction more easily than the non-collapsible ones. If you plan to travel with your poles to your hiking destination, collapsible poles are a must, to fit into your luggage. I'm working on my third pair, top of the line and will see how they hold up. For hiking within driving distance, noncollapsible poles will do the job and can hold up for many years.

Handles: Cork or plastic is the material used for hiking poles. Handle designs vary, some more ergonomic than others. As in choosing shoes, choose the handle that fits you and feels most comfortable in varying temperatures.

Cook Stove

If you want to go ultra light, don't cook and leave the stove at home. If you want more variety in your diet and enjoy a hot drink and a hot meal, bring a stove.

The alcohol stove: Lightweight. The drawback is that it's a more flammable setup and illegal in wildfire-prone wilderness.

The gas canister stove: Lightweight, small, and reasonably priced. My little burner fits folded up in my pot/tall cup. The weight I carry for cooking is the fuel.

The jet boil system: This gas stove with fuel-efficient burner is more expensive and heavier, but saves on fuel, so you're "weighing" the price and weight of the stove against the cost and weight of more canisters.

Water Filtration System

Many choices, many considerations. The bottom line is that you want to have safe drinking water. Picking up an intestinal bug on the trail isn't fun, and the intestinal discomfort can linger for a long time. Here is a list of bacteria and viruses that can make you sick:

Protozoa: This group includes the most commonly feared of all water-borne illnesses: giardia and cryptosporidium. These are single-celled parasitic organisms that cause intense intestinal problems, with symptoms appearing anywhere from 2 days to 2 weeks from ingestion. These organisms can live in cold water for weeks or months at a time. Cryptosporidium has a hard protective outer layer, which makes it resistant to many types of water treatment.

Bacteria: E. coli, which can cause dysentery and campylobacteriosis, as just a few examples, can live in water. These are the easiest pathogens to filter out and treat since they are much larger than viruses.

Viruses: Examples include Hepatitis A and rotavirus. Viruses are not a large threat when hiking and traveling in the United States and Canada, but on international trips, viruses become a much larger concern. Viruses are extremely small, and most filters do not eliminate them.

The choices in filtration systems are plenty. The three factors to juggle are safety, weight, and ease of use, including waiting time after treatment of the water.

Purification drops: Aqua-Mira drops, which contain chlorine and are flavor neutralizing, and are ultra-light. Iodine drops have similar properties if you can handle the taste. These do not treat cryptosporidium, but they do deal with all other problems. I have found that the drops give me sufficiently safe water on the PCT and other West Coast hikes. Waiting time before use of water is 20 minutes.

Steripen: This device treats water with ultra-violet rays. It's small and efficient and treats for cryptosporidium, and there's no waiting time after treating the water. It requires a battery, and the battery runs out fast (6–8 days), so you have to carry extra batteries. I have found this device handy but not reliable. I ended up carrying the drops as backup for when my Steripen failed.

Squeeze or pump filter: The newest on the market is the Sawyer filter, a small lightweight squeeze system you can screw onto a water bottle (you need the right size opening on your bottle). The Sayer is reasonably priced and *safe;* it treats all pathogens, but it's fussy to work with because you have to take your time to squeeze your water through the cartridge. You can screw the smallest version onto your water bottle and drink while sucking the water through the filter. It's handy for day hikes if you don't want to carry much clean water. There are many more water filtration pumping systems, which work if weight isn't an issue because you're at a base camp (a location from which you're taking day hikes) or if you go backpacking for only a few days.

Clothes

Consider *warmth, ventilation, strength, fit, and handy features* when choosing backpacking clothing. Since you'll want to take only a few items of clothing, each one counts and will have to do multiple duty. Your choice of clothes adds to your safety on the trail. Clothes can keep you warm, dry, and protected from sun and nasty scratches, abrasions, or bug bites. Unexpected changes in weather can put you at risk for hypothermia if you're not prepared. A sudden thunderstorm can cause air temperature to drop radically, as this story will tell you.

The weather in the high Sierras is unpredictable, but all reports said to expect occasional thunderstorms in summer that might last an hour. We prepared for rain, but not for long-lasting rain. The summer a friend and I hiked the John Muir Trail in California, it rained every day for almost 3 weeks straight. We were lucky that we caught only the tail end of it and had just a week of rain. We had deliberated over our pack weight and had left the rain pants at home, thinking that our pants would dry fast enough after a sudden rainstorm. When we crossed over Silver Pass, the sunny gorgeous weather became cloudy and the first drops of rain announced a thunderstorm. Shivering in my sun-protection shirt, I added the rain jacket and cover for my pack and hurried down from the pass to get away from open terrain. Within 10 minutes it was hailing and thundering, and the summer world turned into a Christmas card scene.

It was exciting at first, but after two and a half hours of rain, hail, and thunder, the fun was over, torrents of water were turning the trail into a small river, there wasn't a dry spot in sight, and we had to wade with our packs held high through a creek. Even though we were wet and cold and wanted to set up camp to get dry, we couldn't because we were in steep terrain without flat spots. We hiked the whole afternoon with wet shoes, wet feet, and wet legs to keep our blood flowing and stay somewhat warm. At the end of the afternoon the rain stopped, the storm passed, and we were in a spot that was flat enough for setting up camp. Once the tents were up, we could put on dry clothes and climb into our (dry) sleeping bags to get warm again.

Lesson learned: Take full rain gear next time on a long hike, which we did in Washington State, where it always rains. And guess what? It didn't rain, except a few sprinkles one night. We carried the extra weight in an already full pack in 95-degree temperatures up out of the Columbia Gorge! It was so hot that even though we were going slowly I had to lie down on the trail because heat exhaustion made me faint and nauseated. So you see, planning doesn't always pan out.

Protection: For basic protection of the lower part of the body you have the choice of wearing *pants, shorts, or a hiking skirt and socks.* For the upper part of the body, you'll want a short- or long-sleeved shirt or blouse. Many, including men, swear by the coolness and ease of wearing a skirt on the trail. I have met the hiking kilt!

One of my friends, now in her 80s, still hikes, and wears a light dress, her favorite. You can wear a skirt or shorts during summer hiking, but it doesn't work if you need protection from varying temperatures, branches, and rocky outcroppings. Choose your clothing with concern for sun exposure. As we get older, we cannot afford any more sun exposure since we got more than our share in our youth. I cover up as much as possible on sun-exposed trails with hat, fingerless gloves, long-sleeved sun shirt, and long pants.

To protect your face and head, you need a *hat.* The sunhat needs to be light, allow for ventilation, have a tie to tighten under your chin in case of wind, and protect your neck. This hat is not a fashion statement, but serves as a self-care statement. The hat for cold weather needs to be lightweight and warm, and fit under a hooded jacket. To protect you from rain and wind, choose a lightweight, breathable, *rain jacket and pants.*

Gore-Tex is foolproof in wet weather, but new technologies in outdoor apparel appear on the market every year. When you exert yourself in a rain jacket, you sweat, and if the jacket material isn't breathable, condensation will build up inside and get you wet.

Temperature control: Layering is the way to stay warm and cool.

Base layer: One light, short-sleeved shirt, one long-sleeved wicking layer, or a light wool or silk long-sleeved shirt for extra and for sleeping. If you don't care about how you smell, you can sleep in your daytime shirt. Wool wins over polypropylene as far as smell goes, because the polypropylene gets smelly fast. But polypropylene dries faster than wool, so you take your pick. Silk is super lightweight and a good insulator, but not as strong as its polyester counterpart.

Middle layer: This can be an extra base layer long-sleeved shirt, a vest, or a fleece shirt.

Outer layer: The last and important layer is your outer layer for cold mornings and nights, a fleece or down jacket. Again you must weigh the bulk and water resistance of fleece against the lack of water resistance but lighter weight and compactness of down. Rain gear can serve as a temperature control layer as well as protection from wind and rain.

Handy features: My sun shirt has *zippers and vents* on the sides, which can cool me on a hot, sweaty climb. My long-sleeved shirt has *thumbholes* to keep my hands warm and protected. A *chest pocket* allows quick access to lip balm, compass, or any other small device you want to have handy.

Pants with *zip-off legs* are a go-to piece of daily wear. I have a pair with a different-color zipper on each leg zip-off piece, which, after struggling for years to figure out which leg piece goes on which side, is a long-awaited gift. If I had thought of it myself, I could have sewn a little thread to mark the zipper line up. Pockets, many pockets are handy. My trail map for the day slides in and out of my leg pocket many times a day. Zippers and *Velcro tighteners* at the ankle allow for ease of getting in and out of pants while wearing boots or shoes; they also keep out bugs and debris.

First-Aid and Repair Kit

The basic medical kit for day hiking described in Chapter 14 is a good start for backpacking also, with some additions. You cannot prepare for all injuries and medical emergencies, but you can do the basics. I still think how safe we felt hiking for days with a radiologist in the Sierras. He had the ultimate first-aid kit and knew how to use it. We could have had a heart attack, and he would have had a remedy! Here is a list for a wilderness backpacking trip

First-aid kit:

- Ibuprofen and/or aspirin for pain and inflammation.
- A variety of adhesive bandages, including ones for blisters
- An ace wrap for a twisted ankle, a swollen knee, or a sprained wrist
- A sling for a shoulder or arm injury
- A clip for making a tourniquet
- Antibiotic cream
- Personal medication if you use it; add more than enough of a supply for the duration of your trip.

- Depending on the season, a dose of antibiotics in case you get a tick bite
- A salve for dealing with abrasion, dry cracked skin, or irritated areas of your body will be a god-send after a long day on the trail.
- A big clean handkerchief can do wonders for stopping bleeding by using it as a tourniquet. You can also use it as a sling to hold up an arm or to make a splint, so carry at least two on the trail, one for daily wiping, and so on, and one for emergency backup.

Survival/repair kit:

- Matches or a lighter are as much a first-aid item as a survival tool. Keep your matches in a waterproof container, or they'll be useless if you have to wade through a sudden cataract (a large waterfall) and your gear gets wet.
- Sewing supplies, including safety pins
- Duct tape or a clear, strong repair tape
- Sleeping pad repair kit
- Extra shoelaces
- A knife or multi-tool
- Extra batteries

This completes the main components of your outfitting adventure. I will discuss GPS location devices further on. You can find a comprehensive list of items needed for backpacking in the appendix.

Food for the Trail

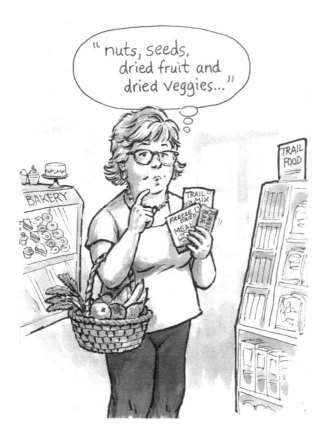

22: Food and Backpacking

I'm a consumer of experiences. I care little for clothes, gadgets, or the latest fad, unless they offer me a new or improved experience. The clothes and gadgets are traveling currency, necessary for me to move around and discover a place I'm heading in life.

I care a lot about food, however, not just as body fuel to enable the moving around, but as experience. A good bouillabaisse in southern France, fresh from the sea with monastery-produced red wine, will forever infuse the palate of my mind. A tangy hot curry in Tamil served in a hall clanging with foreign noises, gives me a ticket to travel back anytime I eat something similar.

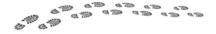

Food on the trail doesn't have to taste like cardboard.

Food on the trail isn't an exciting experience, but one nonetheless, and doesn't have to resemble eating cardboard. What you carry is what you eat. In the comfort of one's home and town, you have access to any kind of food you crave. For the trail, you decide before you leave what you'll eat for a weekend, a week, a month. I give up likes and dislikes for the sake of stamina, lightness of being, and convenience.

Trail Musings

On the trail, I not only feel skin and muscles, the earth's vastness and my smallness, but with the little bags of muesli I pack for breakfast, I bring with me the memory of sitting across from my Swiss lover in a cabin in the snow. When stashing the makings for my cup of Jane— my morning tea, hot, milky and sweet—I pack the benefit of a caffeine-alert mind spilling out ideas as my muscles warm up to the morning trail. Every night, my freeze-dried meals, convenient and measured for calories, give me the choice of revisiting a different place in the world: teriyaki chicken, lasagna, beef Stroganoff, chana masala.

Between morning and night, the food bars fill the holes in the daily food dike on the trail. The modern precursor of the food pill, sugar, fat, and protein combine under different labels, in different colors, with different minor ingredients to pull us to believing we have a choice in taste. Truth: they all taste the same. But they are the fuel in my tank. They leave room for being.

Food as Fuel

Food on the trail means energy. Food is your fuel, the body your engine, the brain the computer that drives the machine.

What do you put in the tank? Ethanol, biofuel, super, or regular? Choices in food are individual. Here are guidelines to help you plan your trail food.

Food for shorter backpack trips can be simple and/or even a gourmet affair. If you go for a few days and don't cook, just do as John Muir did, pack up some bread and water, and you'll survive. I had a backpacking friend who packed an onion, garlic cloves, some leafy greens, a chunk of dense bread, and a few cheeses, and nibbled on her stash throughout the days, never cooking a meal.

I've seen hikers bring their favorite coffeemaker, a glass and boxed wine for afternoon happy hour. I've hauled whole potatoes and canned chili on weekend trips with my children to get them to like backpacking by providing an enticing meal for dinner.

On shorter trips your body can either go with little food or carry more weight, because the shorter duration of the trip leaves you room to play with your desires without putting your survival or performance at risk.

For long trips, food is what will sustain you day after day, mile after mile, so quantity and quality matters. After 2 to 3 weeks on the trail your body will lose its reserves, and if you don't get enough nutrition, you'll run into physical problems and compromise your safety.

A record-setting hiker on the PCT, going by the trail name Anish, broke the record in 2013 (held by Scott Williamson till then) by 4 days. She hiked the length (2650 miles) in 60 days, 17 hours, and 12 minutes. By the time she got to Oregon she was experiencing dizzy spells, leg cramping, and fuzzy vision. She collapsed twice into the dirt. The cause? A shortage of protein while hiking 35 miles a day. By adding lots of protein to her diet she recovered.

The resupply stops are literally that, a resupply for your body and your pack to enable you to do the next stretch. I use a box for each trail section and include everything I'll need at the resupply stop: food, laundry powder, new socks, toilet paper, and so on. Many long-distance hikers resupply their food in towns on the way.

Because not all resupply places stock the items I will want, I mail my resupply boxes to the towns where I'll stop. If I don't need an item when I get to my resupply stop, I leave it behind in the hiker box in the resupply location. In case you're running short or, heaven forbid, your package doesn't arrive, this hiker box can become your salvation for picking up items you need.

Quantity

How much? That depends. To figure out what to take, you must pay attention to calories. The average recommended calorie count in a day for male and female hikers is 2000–4000 calories. For the average 50-plus woman, hiking 8 hours a day, I have found that 1500–2000 calories a day seems to be enough. Remember, food weighs and takes up room in your pack. Again, if you're planning a 3- or 4-day backpacking trip, you can take a more casual approach to quantities.

Forms of Food

Freeze-dried food has been the greatest invention for backpackers. It is light and has a high calorie count for its weight. Freeze-dried breakfasts, lunches, and dinners are available, but it will become costly if all your meals are the freeze-dried kind. I use freeze-dried for dinners and an occasional lunch.

Think in terms of the type of meal: breakfast, lunch, dinner, and snacks. When hiking, it is wise to put food fuel in your tank about every 90 minutes. This provides you with a steady blood sugar level and stamina. Individual differences apply.

Meals

Breakfast

I use my morning energy for walking, thinking, and enjoying the landscape, not for sitting around cooking breakfast. People differ. You may be a slow riser who'd rather loll around awhile before getting started. You may like to hike later in the day and take very little time for dinner.

For breakfast you can consume homemade muesli, a mix of oats, nuts, dried fruit, flaxseed, and milk powder. I pre-package my daily allotment. All I have to do is add (purified) water, let it soak (in a sealed pouch or closed container) while I walk my first stretch of the day, and be ready to chow down after an hour and a half.

It's easy, healthful, and doesn't involve much time; having time to hike in the morning when my energy is high is important to me.

Pop-Tarts are a popular alternative to morning cereal for many hikers, but I find them too sweet and lacking in protein. On more relaxed days I might vary my breakfast fare with a meal of freeze-dried egg and bacon.

My rule of thumb is grains in the morning with some protein, and then more protein as the day progresses, with dinner being my high-protein meal. During the night my body can digest and rebuild.

Each body metabolizes differently. Just realize that you need quick and slow energy provision while hiking, and times for rebuilding your store of energy. Okay, you can always eat just a food bar with a decent amount of protein for breakfast as long as you're getting enough calories.

Lunch

Lunch is a tricky meal. Cooking takes too much time and fuel if you're hiking many miles, bread is bulky, most cheese gets oily, and peanut butter gets boring. I've settled on tortillas or crackers with a filling or topping. Tuna pouches are a great source of protein and weigh little. Note the difference in quality, size, and weight among the various pouches.

I've found sustainably fished tuna in small pouches on sale. When I see a sale, I buy a bunch. For variety, buy salmon. Fish is a good protein and keeps you healthy for the long haul. Don't like fish? Try jerky. Want to eat vegetarian? Eat peanut butter and cheese. Asiago cheese wrapped in cheesecloth will keep for a long time. Freeze-dried fillings, such as fajita wrap filling and chicken salad mix, can work with cold water and add a nice flavored texture to your tortilla. Of course you can eat a food bar for lunch instead.

Dinner

Dinner for me is a freeze-dried meal. It means variety and something warm and tasty after a long day—-my food reward. Several companies make good, sustaining meals. Some are organic, most not. Price varies and, again, be on the lookout for sales. Your local variety store with a camping department might just have a sale for you.

You can try making your own freeze-dried meals. Some of my students tried but found it time consuming and not cost effective. If you have allergies, you might have to follow this route, but I recommend searching for meals that fit your dietary needs among the existing lines first. I add a small bottle of olive oil I can pour on my dinner for added calories. Olive oil boasts a good weight-to-calorie ratio. The tuna pouches can add extra protein to grain-based meals.

Lightweight dried soups add variety in taste and needed salt at the end of sweaty hiking day. In a pinch, dinner can be a food bar, of course.

Snacks

The food bar is the greatest invention for convenience and sustenance. You must wade through the small print on the package to figure out what to put in your body for energy. Sugar? Fat? Protein? I'm a protein junkie, because protein sustains me. Too much sugar creates a blood sugar spike, so I look for bars with 22 grams of protein each. Most bars have 9–11 grams of protein per bar, include sugar and chocolate to make them tasty, and give you a quick burst of energy. You can find recipes to make your own bars. Like them or not, the bars are a lightweight, easy source of food on the trail. I reserve them for snacks and an occasional meal.

If you pay a little more for your bar, you'll get some "real" food value in the form of fat, protein, dried fruits, and some bio-sprouts, flaxseed, and so on. Getting extra nutrients/vitamins added to your bar pays off for the long haul when your body doesn't get much fresh food and might wear down. To add variety to your snacks you can carry trail mix (it's heavy), candy, or chips (if you want crunch in your diet). I save my appetite for tasty foods for the resupply days when I'm off the trail and can wander in the world of grocery stores and restaurants.

Gathering Your Food and Packing

For multiday trips, decide how much food you'll need for the length of your trip (plus some extra in case of delays) and put it in plastic bags or carry it in its original packaging. If you use freeze-dried food, you can leave it in the handy pouches or repack it in less bulky packaging. If you plan to cook, you can use your pot to cook your meal or just to heat water for your freeze-dried dinner and bring one of the handy pouches to rhydrate the food, leaving your pot clean.

For long trips, if you are particular about what you eat, create your daily necessary meals and multiply by the number of days you'll be on the trail between resupply stops, with extra in case of unwanted delays. On the John Muir Trail we hiked with a man whose resupply box didn't arrive twice. There weren't any good grocery stores at the resupply spots, so he resupplied himself from the hiker box. It wasn't his first choice (he was a man who liked his wine and peanuts at the end of a long day), but he survived and kept on hiking.

You'll develop your own system for packing your food as you start hiking longer stretches. I repack my freeze-dried food in small plastic bags and take one of the handy pouches for dinner and one for breakfast rehydrating. I create a breakfast, lunch, dinner, and snack bag, so I can easily find the individual items I need for the day when on the trail. I've gone from one container for peanut butter or honey to individual pouches; they're less messy and the contents come out more easily when cold mornings have hardened the contents. Note that individual packaging of meals creates more trash you have to carry out. I now buy biodegradable plastic baggies, carry them out, and wash and reuse them until they are no longer usable. You'll want to be the kind of person who carries her trash out once you've spent time in the beauty of the wilderness and seen what people leave.

Once you have your food figured out, the (not so) fun part of trying to fit everything into your pack begins. When you weigh your full pack, you'll most likely find out it's heavier than you'd realized. Then the nitty-gritty decision making starts of what to leave behind.

23: Staying Safe for the Distance

A friend and I were on a multiday backpacking trip in the mountains of southern Oregon, a forested area. I had hiked the trail several times before and was familiar with it. We followed its rise along a river and hiked up to the bottom of a steep climb to reach a cirque where we camped for the night. The next morning, we started a loop around the cirque at about 6800 feet elevation. From the trail, we spotted the top of a small mountain (Aspen Butte) overlooking the cirque and decided to hike there to enjoy a 360-degree view of the area. We left our packs at the trail and climbed for 20 minutes on brushy and rocky terrain to reach the wonderful all-around view at the top.

After enjoying the view, we hiked down. There was no trail, so the direction down was a guess, but we figured we couldn't be far off. We ended up on the trail but not where our packs were. We had to decide if we should turn left or right to find them. It took hiking in the wrong direction quite a way before I realized we were way past the area where we might have left our packs, so we backtracked and eventually found our packs again. A GPS device could have helped us. Carrying our packs on our backs up the mountain would have been a wiser solution. It seemed so innocent to take a little side jaunt up the mountain. Everything turned out okay, but it might not have.

To track where you are and stay on the trail on long-distance hikes, you need a topo map, a compass, and a GPS guidance device. If your GPS fails, if you run out of battery power, you will want a printed map for backup. Topo maps will offer you an overview of the day's terrain, whereas the GPS device offers a more detailed update of where you are as you move along the trail or if you find yourself off-trail.

The compass can help you if your GPS fails and you need to go off-trail to hike out. My story of going off-trail should serve as a warning. If you have to go off-trail because you need to get back sooner than planned, have a compass and know how to use it. Orienting yourself in canyons can be tricky; canyons and ridges can look the same, and if you think you can cut across to catch the trail on the other side again, you might be in for a surprise.

Topo Map

Before you head out on the trail, learn to read a topo map: green means forest, spotted green and white means you're near the tree line, white means rocks and no trees, and so on. Learn that the contour lines follow elevation lines, so you can see if the trail is going up steeply, gradually, or down. A topo map covering the length of your trail gives you an overview, and for multiday hiking, will help you plan your route and find alternate connecting trails and trailheads. With a topo map, for example, you'll be able to see when you will be in the shade of trees, or on exposed terrain. This can be important if you are hiking in the hot season and want to stay cooler while going uphill.

If you plan to hike the PCT, free downloadable topo maps are available online (Halfmile Maps).

For 2- or 3-day backpacking trips, a guidebook of the destination area may be enough if you are familiar with the terrain and you stay on a known trail and follow the posted signs. It will tell you the elevation, length and difficulty of a hike, and the seasons when the trail is accessible. It will usually give you a simple drawing of the trail and its environment and the rivers you'll cross or hike along, as well as the passes and mountaintops you'll reach. But if you want to have the flexibility of altering your route, or extending your trip, a topo map is very helpful for on-the-trail planning.

The Compass

The compass has long been a go-to Boy Scout tool for finding your way. With GPS devices so available, use of the compass has declined, and the need for a compass is unlikely when hiking well-marked trails. A compass doesn't weigh much, so keep one in your pack, and use it to brush up on your skill, so you'll have it in case you get lost and don't have a GPS device to guide you back to familiar territory.

GPS

Halfmile Maps offers a free PCT app for your phone, which will give you via satellite in text format your location in coordinates and your mileage point on the trail, indicating distances to important landmarks, campsites, water sources, trail access, and resupply points along the way. Guthook offers a similar app with 3D maps, marking campsites, water sources and side trails as if reading a marked up topo map. Guthook charges a subscription fee to run the app, and charges you for the maps you download.

Not all trails are as well documented as the PCT and AT (Appalachian Trail). You need GPS guidance when you go places that are poorly documented, such as the Continental Divide Trail running from the Mexican border to Canada across the Continental Divide, or the Hayduke Trail in Utah, or when you have to traverse snowfields for a good distance and can't see the trail

On one of my recent hikes we encountered a snowfield. We followed footsteps in the snow which led us higher and higher on the ridge. I had hiked this trail in the past without snow, and knew that we were too high up to be on the trail. By using my GPS app, I could steer us in the general direction of the trail while choosing a safe crossing around tree wells and up steep snowbanks.

To keep track of your location on or off a trail, you'll need a GPS device or a general GPS app such as the Gaia app, to let you see where you're going, let you keep track of your location and find the trail in case you lose it. Both a GPS device and the Gaia app require you to download a map of your destination area before you go out into the wilderness.

GPS Contact

For contact and emergency airlifting these are the two most-used devices:

SPOT is a safety GPS tracking device for messaging loved ones and provides tracking for those who need to be informed about where you are. It will show interested ones at home, via a pre-composed message and GPS link, where you are and where you have walked on a particular day. It doesn't show you a map of the area you're in, but the link gives readers at home a Google Earth map of your location. It has an SOS button to push in case an airlift is needed, and a special message button if you want to be picked up at a location by your support person.

InReach is a satellite phone device that allows the user to connect with the populated world via text message. In case of emergency the user can text back and forth with rescuers to provide specific information about the emergency and receive notice of rescue efforts. There is a monthly fee, which ends up being more expensive in a year than the yearly fee for the SPOT device.

Mapping Your Hike

To plan for your safety on your hike, a hiking plan offers you and your support team a tool to know where you are likely to be on any given day. Mapping out daily mileage considering the difficulty of the terrain helps with planning for a successful hike. Even though your daily plan may change because of trail and personal circumstances, having a general plan is a way to keep track for those supporting you and keeps you from running out of food before you get to your next resupply location.

To make a hiking plan, you need to note mileage, water sources, camping spots and elevations. Elevations indicate the pace you may be able to set for a stretch of the trail. Available camping sites and water sources will determine where you will stop for the night. From training before your hike you know how many miles you can do comfortably in a day. Use this to gauge your average daily mileage for the trail, taking the elevation into account. For most well-known, long-distance trails, elevation profiles are available either in a guidebook or online, posted there by someone who has taken the time to map out the elevations for their own use. An elevation profile will plot the valleys and mountaintops from point A to point B on a graph. The height is shown on the vertical coordinate and the distance in miles on the horizontal coordinate. This is a useful depiction of the difficulty of your terrain.

A lot of peaks and valleys over a short distance means days full of climbing and descending. For the type of terrain—rocky, brush, or forest duff—you'll want to check a guidebook or your topo map. You'll need the elevation profile to plan how far you can hike in a day and where you want to camp. If possible do your climbing in the earlier part of the next day when you're fresh. Avoid camping on a high mountain pass; weather can be an issue up high. Climbing in the early part of your day is not always possible, but it's something to strive for when planning your hiking days.

Adjust your hiking plan if needed when you encounter the reality of the trail. On one of my long hikes with trainees, we had to lower our average daily mileage to accommodate a severe case of blisters. Our daily GPS message to our support person with our location let them know our pace had slowed.

Support and Backup

Once you've created a daily hiking plan with the help of your maps and elevation profile, give this plan to your main support person(s). Your support person can be a partner, family member, or friend, or several people willing to be your backup in case you need supply packages sent to your resupply points or someone to come bail you out if you want to leave the trail. The plan will let them know where you'll be on the trail.

Make a daily check-in plan with your support person(s)—include as many people as your device allows—by using either your GPS device or satellite phone to send information with your location. You can also call your support person(s) when you have phone access to let them know of your progress on the trail and how you're holding up. Unless you're experienced in using a GPS device to help you navigate cross-country, stay with your hiking plan and on the trail, where you'll meet others who can be of help when needed.

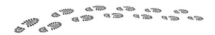

A daily check-in plan with support people is a bridge to safety while on the trail.

The Hiking Community

Besides relying on maps and GPS devices, your fellow hikers on your hikes are your community and your support. Hikers greet each other, exchange information, and offer help when needed. You may save someone's life by telling them that the next water source has dried up or that the trail is closed because of fire; they may save you from an uncomfortable night by telling you about a constant howling wind at the camping spot near the pass.

Once when I was hiking solo, I entered a trail leading to Jefferson Park in Oregon near Mount Jefferson and I saw a sign posted on the trail. It was a picture of a man in his mid-50s above the words, "Man lost. Please report if you have seen this man." While wondering what could have happened, I looked up ahead and saw a snowfield.

As I climbed south toward the snowfield I had to cross to get to the pass leading into the park and I met a north-bound hiker. We talked awhile and exchanged information, and I asked him whether it was easy to find the trail in the snow, since I did not have a GPS mapping device (I had my SPOT, cell phone, and trail maps).

He told me he had just come across the snowfield and to follow his footsteps in the snow, keeping the crooked outcropping of the pass, which we could see in the distance, on my left. When I entered the snowfield, I clearly saw his sunken boot marks in the snow. I followed them, but at some point it was difficult to differentiate his footsteps from the cupping of the snow that occurs as it melts and freezes. I lost his trail, kept my eye on the outcropping, found what looked like another set of footsteps going in the right direction, and luckily came to the snowless pass.

From the pass there wasn't a visible trail down, just a boulder field. I could make out a lake way below, one I recognized from my map as Russell Lake, around which the trail circled. So I set out, scooting myself down-slope from boulder to boulder with my pack on my back, not daring to jump and hurt my knees.

As I sat to rest, I heard a heavy whirr of a helicopter over my head. I had to duck because the noise and wind were so intense, and three men jumped from the sky and scrambled over to me.

"You're a woman," they exclaimed with disappointment.

"Yes, what's the problem with that?" I said.

"We're looking for a man in his mid-50s, with an orange pack and beige hat, and you have orange on your pack and have a beige hat. We're sorry if we scared you."

The search-and-rescue guys, which is what they turned out to be, were looking for the lost man on the notices. I asked them where the trail was, and they suggested that if I followed them, I would find it.

I couldn't keep up with them though, for they were like strong mountain goats jumping and running down the mountain. I followed the general direction and found the trail without difficulty.

I heard through the trail grapevine later that the lost man had left his party to take some pictures of the snowfield, planning to catch up with his party afterward. He was never found; weeks of searching did not bring him back.

The lesson to learn from this story: do not wander off alone on dangerous terrain (snowfields, crevasses, slides). If you have to cross snowy areas of the trail, have a device that can send out your location if you have an accident. The information I got from a fellow hiker when crossing the snowfield provided me with a safe crossing. I was glad I'd asked for help. The thought of the man somewhere lost on that same field kept me on alert.

Section IV

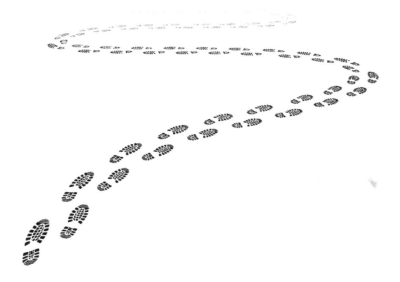

Frequently Asked Questions

1. Wild Animals

"What about bears and cougars?" is the first thing people ask me about my long hikes in the wilderness. I tell them that accidents from animal attacks are minimal; car accidents are far more frequent. Animal danger does depend on where you go. In the western United States, bears are common and cougars do roam but there is safety in numbers on the trail, because both bears and cougars avoid people, especially noisy groups. I have seen bears from a distance, but they disappeared pretty quickly. I've learned that cougar sightings are rare, since they are stalkers if they are in attack mode. Cougars attack single hikers, not groups, and if they attack, they are more likely to go after children more than full-grown humans.

Large numbers of people in the wilderness can actually attract bears, as do the campers in Yosemite National Park. California bears are after food, so putting food in a bear canister away from your camp will deter them.

Other parts of the world have their own dangers. How about getting in the middle of a yak fight in the Himalayas? When I trekked in Ladakh, I saw yaks grazing at high altitude. They seemed as docile as cows. One afternoon when we had stopped early below a snowy pass, I came out of my bright orange tent to go take a bath in the nearby river and found myself 6 feet away from two snorting, bucking 200-pound males, who had locked horns and were pulling each other back and forth in a wild display of male testosterone. No female yak in sight. Was it my orange tent that had set them off? The ground was shaking under their hooves. I didn't know what they would do if I moved and they noticed me, so I stood there frozen, hoping they would take their aggression out on each other, not on me.

After a wild 15-minute show, they let go of each other's horns, lumbered off, and resumed their grazing. I took a wide berth around them to get to the river. I never looked at docile yaks the same way again.

In the desert and hot parts of the wilderness there are snakes. Watch where you put your feet when you climb over a rock or a log, for snakes might lie just on the other side, warming themselves. They seek warm spots at night when temperatures drop. Keep your tent closed so a snake won't get in when you're not watching.

While hiking in the wilderness use your common sense. Don't attract animals by leaving food lying around. Use a bear-proof sack and hang your food, or a bear-proof canister to stash your food away from your camp. Stay on trails, make noise when you spot a wild animal, and make yourself big by raising your arms with hiking poles in the air.

Reports of bear attacks on clearly laid-out trails in Yellowstone National Park have increased, and you want to take special precautions when you hike there. If a bear attacks, roll up into a ball on the ground, protect your head and freeze. If the bear thinks you're dead, it may lose interest. Carrying bear spray may make you feel safer, but from the reports of bear attacks, it all happens so fast that bear spray hasn't time to come to the rescue. To inform yourself about animal danger, contact the local Forest Service in the area you're planning to visit for details.

2. Injuries

Basic first-aid knowledge is a must for being out in the wilderness. Your medical kit should be able to help you take care of minor injuries. A fall on the trail can cause a sprain, scrape, or bruise. Ice-cold water, snow, or an icepack can soothe a sprain. Anti-inflammatories can help with pain and allow you to hike on. If you're lucky, other hikers will come along and help you.

Decide whether you're in a place from which you can be rescued. Are you visible to others, either from the sky or from a nearby trail? If you're not visible, move to a more visible place, if possible. Look around and figure out where you can create shelter for yourself so you can stay warm and protected for the time it takes for help to arrive. Wear or display bright contrasting colors so you may be seen more easily. If it makes sense to draw the attention of people nearby, make the SOS signal on your whistle—three short blasts, three long blasts, three short blasts—and repeat this signal at regular intervals. Use the SOS button on your safety device to broadcast your location and alert a rescue mission.

If you're injured or lost to a degree that prevents you from hiking out, stop where you are, stay calm, and assess your situation. Taking the time to make a well-thought-out plan for safety is better than rushing off in an unknown direction seeking help.

3. Hygiene.

Basic cleanliness prevents problematic issues on the trail. Since rashes can develop in sensitive areas if you don't keep clean, wash when you can, using water from a stream, a lake, or a spring.

Bring a washrag (a bandana or any piece of soft cloth dedicated for the purpose) and non-polluting soap.

Change out your socks and underwear regularly to prevent blisters and rashes.

For cleaning after "bathroom" use, you can use toilet paper or antiseptic wipes, but leaving toilet paper or wipes behind, buried or not, creates wilderness pollution, since animals may dig it up or rain may unearth it.

Instead, carry out your toilet paper or wipes, or use a small bottle with a spray top as a "bidet" to rinse after moving your bowels. Use a rag to wipe after urinating, which can be washed, *away from the water source!* Carry a small bottle of hand sanitizer to clean your hands if no water is nearby to wash your hands.

Be cautious about sharing food and gear with other hikers. Bacterial diseases get passed on easily when hand-washing possibilities are minimal.

4. Safe Drinking Water

If you hike more than a day, you will have to rely on natural water sources for your drinking water, such as streams, lakes, and springs. As I suggested in the section about gear, bring a filter to purify your water and avoid nasty intestinal diseases. Check water sources before you go on your hike to calculate how much water is available and how much you will have to carry. Remember the rule of thumb is 1 liter of water for 4 miles of hiking. If you end up in a "dry" camp (no access to water nearby), you will have to carry enough from your last water source to make it through the night (dinner and breakfast). Carry extra foldable water bottles if water is scarce on the trail.

Section V

The Art of Living After 50

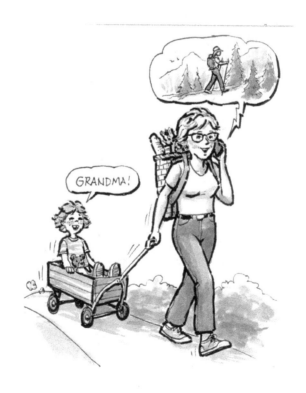

24: Success and the Art of Living

We live in a world where success is measured by numbers and rankings: in sports, finances, acquisitions, best-seller lists, and brands. We no longer measure success by the health and happiness of the family we create, the land we cultivate, or the peace deals we strike in a lifetime.

Women have traditionally been less acknowledged in public for their success. The saying "Behind every successful man stands a woman" indicates the secondary role women have played in politics, business, and government. Which woman anymore wants to have her success measured by the number of children she has raised?

Women are fighting to change their role in society, but for women it's an extra burden to achieve success. As Ginger Rogers said, "I can do everything the man does, only backwards and in high heels."

To be successful, a woman has to *look* successful, which means young—younger than her age. When I see the Botox marks on an older stateswomen's face, I feel sorry that she has to subject herself to this treatment to have a chance for success in her campaign.

Women know success in life can come in small moments: in an interview that lands you a job, a soufflé that comes out of the oven high and fluffy, or a walk around the block after surgery. As Oprah Winfrey said, "Step out of the history that is holding you back. Step into the new story you are willing to create."

Success is the moment you experience a lift of spirit, whether or not that moment is recognized by others. Successful living is made up of many such moments, strung together into a feeling of confidence, a feeling of *I can*. Individuals experience that lift of spirit differently, but the endpoint of autonomous strength and empowerment is the same. Repeated failures, repeated losses, and traumas all erode our confidence in living.

When I was dealing with the trauma of repeated loss, I wanted to escape this life. I remembered a barren place in the Himalayas I had seen in pictures and decided I wanted to journey there. So I went for a walk, a trek in the mountains. On this trek I experienced the daily simplicity of walking, breathing, and being able to tackle the elements. As my body moved along the miles on the trail, I found myself again. I gained the confidence that no matter what happened, I always had that place inside me that I call self-belonging.

My motivation initially was simply to walk away from the life I didn't want to endure. I thought I could disappear, get away from the world, and maybe become a Buddhist hermit in a cave. I wanted to leave my depression behind. My body was healthy enough to enable me to keep moving until a new horizon came into view.

When things are miserable, you have two choices: you can stay in the misery or you can leave. Either way takes energy, but staying in the misery is the road to decline, whereas trying something new might be the road to success. The beginning of a new life can literally happen one step at a time.

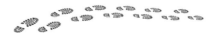

Becoming a walking woman plants the feeling of being successful deep inside you.

Becoming a walking woman is one of those small successes that won't make the news, won't earn you a medal, and may not even get noticed or valued by your family. Becoming a walking woman plants the feeling of being successful deep inside you. It nourishes conviction: as long as you can make a change and stick with it, you have life left in you. Change is truly the only constant you can count on in life. Living with and accepting change is the artful way to live.

Trail Musings

Every day I walked, every day I completed another stretch without pain or accident, the trust in my body grew. In my mind I heard, "I can do this, my body will let me do this." Joyful in my capable body, I started each day refreshed. A body that walks affirms living. A body that walks gives joy. Even tired walking at the end of a day was propelled by the motion of the day, the momentum of rhythmic motion.

The steep mountainsides, some of them bare, some covered by trees, rose above me and fell off below me. The trail was narrow. One step wrong, and I could lose my balance and roll. My stomach did a somersault when I looked down. I could see my body swaying with the pack and being pulled down, down, bumping against trees, branches, and rocks, landing in a snow patch somewhere. Then I looked up and ahead. I wouldn't let that happen.

The flat ground of my campsite that evening felt like an overwhelming expanse. Feeling its spacious support, I slept deeply and well that night. As the days and mountainsides rolled by, I became alert, shed the terror, and walked easily on the narrow, steep trails. I discovered the "RAM" in the computer of my brain. I had accessed the power of confidence through walking.

I dreamed seemingly significant dreams early every morning. I wrote them down in my journal. I interpreted them over breakfast or during my first stretch of walking when my mind was still embedded in the associative sleep-wake state. From my dreams, I figured out what was important in my life at this time. They clarified what I needed to focus on when I returned to my regular life. I needed to keep working to make eventual retirement more comfortable, but I could simplify my daily living and create more spaciousness on my days off.

Regular life. I hadn't been thinking about it. I was in a new "regular" life, and absorbed in the routine of it.

I had no mirror. I could not see myself unless I bent over the water surface of a lake or peered into the black screen of my phone, turned off as it was. I didn't know what I looked like. I had lost a sense of my age. I was just who I was. I met another woman on the trail who looked older than I perceived myself to be. After we had talked for a while, I asked her age. It was the same as mine. Did I look like her? I realized that we think of ourselves as being of a certain age, with a certain confidence, a certain beauty because we live with reflections of ourselves at every turn. I liked the freedom that came with being me, without age, without physical attractiveness, with just the strength in my legs and my back and my kindness to whomever I met to determine who I was for the day.

25: Walking to Enhance Your Spirit

"If you are ready to leave father and mother—if you have paid your debts, and made your will, and settled all your affairs, and are a free [wo]man—then you are ready for a walk . . . No wealth can buy the requisite leisure, freedom, and independence which are the capital in this profession . . . It requires a direct dispensation from Heaven to become a walker."

Such was Thoreau's challenge. Heaven and its dispensation aside, he understood that becoming a walker is a spiritual endeavor. You can't become a walker without confronting your state of mind. As we age, our state of mind determines our happiness. Diane von Furstenberg agrees when she says, "You are the one that possesses the keys to your being. You carry the passport to your own happiness."

To understand how the connection between mind and body works, let's delve into the practice of mindfulness training, a training derived from Eastern spiritual practices.

Travelers to Asia in the 1970s came in contact with meditation practices that they then introduced to the West. Over time, the value of these spiritual practices for daily living was recognized, and studies followed, documenting the outcome of mindfulness training. MBSR, Mindfulness Based Stress Reduction, as it is called, is an 8-week program developed by Dr. Jon Kabat-Zin and medical and psychology students at the University of Massachusetts Medical School in the early 1990s.

Training in mindful living has gone mainstream in the last decades. Ever since scientific studies have demonstrated its effectiveness in reducing stress and increasing focused awareness, the medical world has incorporated this training into dealing with illness. Even the government uses it as part of their military training as a tool for dealing with the stress of war and for helping the mind to be more resilient.

The value of mindfulness for our physical health, resilience, and peace of mind is now an accepted fact. If you haven't practiced earlier in your life, it's not too late to add this technique to your daily mental hygiene. Most mindfulness training is done as a sitting exercise. Zen Buddhists, however, developed walking meditation centuries ago. This form of meditation develops awareness as you move (slowly) with attention.

I'm a longtime practitioner of mindfulness training, the sitting kind. But on my longer hikes, when I had to move slowly under a heavy pack, I discovered the mindfulness aspect of hiking. The attention required for traversing uneven terrain, for slipping into a rhythm and adopting a pace you can maintain for long stretches, parallels the attention a meditator develops by focusing on the breath going in and out. It doesn't matter what you focus on, though; the capacity to stay focused will serve you when you are dealing with the unpleasantries of life, be they the steep terrain, the heaviness of a pack, or the vicissitudes of daily living. If you can stay calm and detached, or at least somewhat detached—keeping your equanimity, as it is called in meditation training—when pain enters your body or your mind, you will suffer less and you will build a calmer, more stable mind for dealing with future pain.

We will suffer in life. The Western way of dealing with suffering has been to avoid it by making things pleasant and easier, by distraction. And haven't we done a great job in the West of creating our creature comforts? The Eastern way has been to face suffering head-on while knowing it will pass. This stoic acceptance of the unpleasant things in life, however, often translates into a lag in the development of new products, new medical interventions, and scientific discoveries, which could prevent suffering.

There is a middle way. Without enduring more suffering than is necessary, accepting the pains and stress of life, such as illness, loss, and misfortunes, without over-reacting to them creates a strong mind, a mind that is at the owner's command, a mind that, in its dispassionate observing, is free to develop compassion and love for humankind, for the preciousness of life.

If performed properly, and with awareness, daily walking, seasonal hiking, and long-distance trekking are a prescription for the spiritual training of mindfulness. Since there are indications that mindfulness alters our bodies on a cellular level, mindful walking will have a positive effect on our health. Daily walking is your daily meditation, seasonal hikes are your short retreats from life to strengthen body and mind, and long hikes are the long retreats for training the mind and cleansing deep disturbances, both physical and mental.

In Cheryl Strayed's book *Wild*, she tells the story of hiking the PCT to get away from her use of drugs, her grief over her mother's death, and the general mess of her life. On the trail, she faces all the mind-sets that have caused the suffering in her life. On the trail, she works through and changes those mind-sets. Her hike becomes a training in mindfulness.

Not everyone begins a long hike because her life is a mess. Not everyone is intent on developing mindfulness. But if you go out for whatever reason, and you pay attention, you will discover the state of mind meditators seek, a state of mind induced by a healthy blood flow, infused with endorphins, and a breathing pattern that better regulates your functioning both of limbs and of organs. You will discover that you feel better and are becoming healthier.

If your walking isn't too bogged down by physical or mental suffering or distracted by being plugged into an electronic device, the beauty of the vistas will affect you, you will notice the patterns of nature, and you will develop an enhanced awareness of your surroundings away from distractions. Your attention will zero in on a leaf color, the shape of a rock in its simple beauty, its place in the whole of things. Without trying, you will develop an appreciation for all things around you, a love for nature, which will foster compassion and kindness toward all.

Back in the early 1990s the Japanese Ministry of Agriculture, Forestry and Fisheries coined the term Shinrin-yoku, "forest bathing," a practice that encourages people to immerse themselves in nature to boost the immune system, reduce stress, and develop mindfulness. It's fast becoming a prescription for health in the West. Thoreau again:

I am alarmed when it happens that I have walked a mile into the woods bodily, without getting there in spirit. In my afternoon walk, I would fain forget all my morning occupations and my obligations to Society. But it sometimes happens that I cannot easily shake off the village. The thought of some work will run in my head and I am not where my body is—-I am out of my senses. In my walks I would fain return to my senses. What business do I have in the woods, if I am thinking of something out of the woods?

By becoming a Walking Woman, you can experience the joy of having a body. As I describe in *NOW, a book of moments*:

I walk away, I walk on, grateful to have a body that serves me. A body that supports and contains the endless gyrations of a mind over-stimulated by a society that cannot say 'enough,' that can't say 'NO' to the flood of information and artificial stimulation it produces. I will not walk away from society forever, live as a hermit.

However, camping at the base of Mt Hermit gave me thought about the steady stillness a mountain produces. A stillness I crave from deep within. I am glad I have that craving. I am glad it takes me to great heights and long walks where I can experience that stillness in myself, step by step. The transformation that took place on this trip, is not a transformation of my being; it is a transformation of finding and returning to my original being, my belonging self. That quiet emptiness I take across the pass with me, into the life, which is now.

At a time in life when we think our bodies are failing us, when we fear gravity is taking over and our bodies begin to droop in unintended places, when we disconnect from our bodies because they don't give us as much pleasure, we can reconnect with ourselves in a deeper way by using our bodies as vehicles for joy and connectedness as we walk.

The aliveness we feel as we take a walk or a hike or spend weeks in the wilderness is an aliveness that changes us on a cellular level. It changes our brains and how we experience our world. For longtime meditators the expanded state of mind, the increased activity of the frontal cortex (which helps in making good decisions and living an intentional life), and the reduced activity in the amygdala (the center of stress and emotional reactivity in the brain) become the new baseline, the new ordinary state of mind. Researcher Joshua Grant studied pain sensitivity in Zen meditators and found a "pain-lessening effect," . . . "a permanent change in their perception."

When you make walking a part of your life, you will move your baseline activity and wellbeing to a higher level, resulting in improved health and deeper satisfaction. You will discover benefits similar to those enjoyed by experienced meditators. The often-noted agelessness of experienced meditators and spiritual teachers might not just be a result of experiencing less stress.

Grant also found that their engagement in regular exercise and endurance exercise caused an increased activity of telomerase, a ribonucleoprotein that adds protective sequences to the end of the telomeres region of chromosomes, thereby protecting the end of chromosomes from DNA damage, and decreased senescent marker P16 (markers of cellular aging in the blood). In other words the study showed that regular exercise had triggered an anti-aging process.

Walking can serve as a vehicle not only for health and equanimity, but as a way of feeling connected. As we age, the chances of becoming disconnected from our loved ones increase. The dire image of a lonely, old, and depressed woman does not have to haunt us, even if we lose our partner to death or divorce, or our children to the world. We can replace the connectedness to loved ones we developed earlier in life with a general sense of connectedness. This is a blessing awaiting us. We merely have to seek it.

Trail Musings

Diamond Peak: Long ago, before the last ice age, she rose, pushed out by volcanic eruption, a painful birth, crags sticking up like unruly rocky hair in all directions. When young, she was hard to touch. Time wore away her spiky hair, a few small eruptions followed, and she became a beauty, lying there, her snow-covered breasts exposed. I watch her from a half-day's walking distance, my feet dangling in a warm lake fed by the river coming down from her slopes. I am in love with this day, this sight. Goodness gathers in this bright moment. I have followed the trail, maybe foolishly so, and now I drink the beauty. I will work my muscles to keep up with her heights, even though I fear her moods, as she can turn her weather on a dime. She is here and I am open to her presence. All I have to do is commit myself to the trail, walk, and be aware.

In drunken hopefulness, I sleep and wake early to climb along her side. High up under the snow the clefts between her rocky surface form gullies filled with glacial milk. Below I drink from the ice-cold pools among the soft moss and fern hair. A wind stirred up by the warm morning sun cools the sweat already dripping down my back. Higher still, the trees are shrinking, becoming more sparse. Flowery meadows make way for yellow pockets of ground-up calcium basalt held in place by sprigs of grass, a dune landscape at 7000 feet.

I become a child again, as I once was, five steps ahead of my family climbing those dunes eager for the day of sun and sea waiting on the other side.

What lies on the other side of her slopes? The empty trail lies behind me as I climb higher and higher. I don't look back. I don't want to know the emptiness, not now. I am climbing the slopes of this peak, and I let myself be pulled over her shoulder to what lies beyond, another mile, another day, another mountain, another opportunity to live life.

As we age, we can become an inspiring example of living life gracefully and fully, by adopting simple, available practices that will enhance the quality of life. A woman who is radiant because she enjoys her life becomes a magnet for others, and she will find herself part of a community that adds to her sense of belonging and connectedness. The knife cuts two ways in this case. Remember the story of the woman by the creek in the beginning of this book? A younger, not so happy woman was drawn to the older, vibrant women to ask advice. The title of Crone can have a positive connotation, someone with radiance and wisdom, a "crowned" person.

Women who pay attention to the self are not being selfish, but self-enhancing. As they say during the safety talk on the airplane, "Put on your own oxygen mask first. You cannot help someone else if you are not breathing." Find out how you can enhance yourself through mindful walking and hiking. Find out how you can become a confident "enhanced" person, an inspiration for others.

The growth forces that earlier in our life helped us become attractive women and nurturers of family and community can now be expressed through us in artful living, the "crowning" (crone-ing) of our existence as women. Rather than withering away, we can take care of our bodies and let our spirits shine. When the daily nurturing of a family, a business, or a profession falls away, many women find the time to create by channeling life energy and turning this energy into visible, audible, and experiential forms of sharing. As women age, they can share their life energy and create a legacy of beauty for those around them and those who will come after.

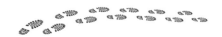

Walking for health and awareness then becomes a walking into the light.

26: Walking Home to Myself

Trail Musings

I am walking south on a narrow path winding its way through the endless forest of my home state. It feels as if the trees keep coming my way, like soldiers, an army, in a march for occupation, and I feel small, vulnerable. Some days I see the trees as a forest of faceless people walking the street of a big city. Faceless people with eyes inward, their mind connected with thoughts, a phone, or the person talking next to them.

I walk and the trees keep coming. The square holes in the bark where the PCT signs have been removed, gape like an open mouth calling out, "Hey, that was my face you just took away." Every couple of hundred feet, another open mouth shows itself, the bark grow-ing scar tissue all around the exposed epithelium.

On some stretches the trees are dressed alike, tall, straight grain of bark tunneling upward. The closeness of the trees kills the undergrowth, forbids the fancy, lacy, lacy fern, the huckleberry, the flowers, the color. Gray-brown bark matches the duff under the fallen ones, the broken dead ones, the disintegrating ones. The trees in their dark suits stand watch over the graveyard.

On other stretches the trees stand apart enough to form twirling green dresses with their branches. Dappled light paints shadows and yellow patterns on the perky leaves of the grasses, the star clusters of pink mountain laurel lining the edge of the trail. The light on the mosaic of moss and stone on the path taps a silent symphony of eternal beauty.

I enter a battlefield, strewn with the remnants of the war between trees and fire. The dead ones stand naked, scorched, black arms reaching in a helpless gesture to the sky. Rain and snow will rot these hands; heat and wind will dry them and make them fall. I walk in burnt forest long after. Grass sparks the black earth green again. Fireweed holds its magenta crown against the sun-bleached wood of the tree stumps, the new color scheme of aging. Alpine huckleberries offer their small tart taste when I sit down and let the morning sun warm me.

Around me loss is holding hands with beauty. I can no longer feel sorry for myself over the loss of a great love. Life is in my hands, beauty in my eyes. I am walking home to myself, and the trees keep coming.

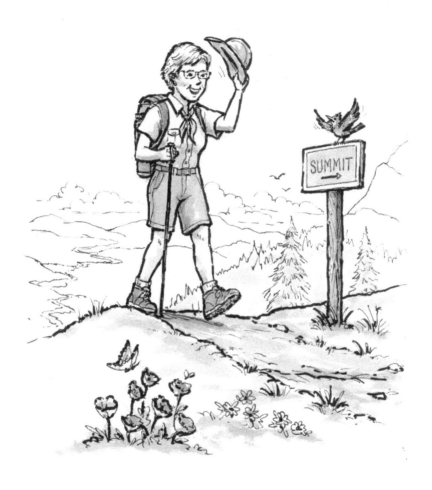

Congratulations!

You've finished the first step toward becoming a walking woman. I hope you'll help more women take that step by sharing *Walking Gone Wild* on your social media accounts.

How about a review? I would greatly appreciate it if you would share what you think about *Walking Gone Wild* with a review on a blog or the online bookstores.

Now take step two: Go for a walk. Set a walking goal for yourself.

One more step: join the WalkingWomen50-plus community. Our Facebook page is https://www.facebook.com/walkingwomen50plus/, and our Twitter handle is @dami97520.

I hope to see you there!

Happy walking,

Dami

More from Fuze Publishing

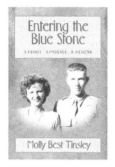

Entering the Blue Stone by Molly Best Tinsley

The General battles Parkinson's; his wife manifests a bizarre dementia. Their grown children embrace what seems a solution—an upscale retirement community. Between laughter and dismay, discover what shines beneath catastrophe: family bonds, the dignity of even an unsound mind, and the endurance of the heart. *Memoir*

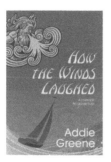

How the Winds Laughed by Addie Greene

When Addie Greene and her young husband take on the "great adventure" of circumnavigation in a 28-foot boat, a succession of catastrophes demands that she become the driving force in carrying them forward and safely home. *Memoir*

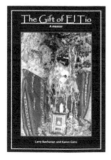

The Gift of El Tio by Larry Buchanan and Karen Gans

When a world-renowned geologist discovers an enormous deposit of silver beneath a remote Quechua village in Bolivia, he unknowingly fulfills a 450-year-old prophecy that promised a life of wealth for the villagers.

Memoir

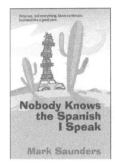

Nobody Knows the Spanish I Speak by Mark Saunders

High-tech couple from Portland, Oregon, emigrates with large dog and ornery cat to San Miguel de Allende, in the middle of Mexico. Their well-intentioned cluelessness makes for mayhem and nonstop laughs. *Memoir*

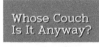

Whose Couch Is It, Anyway? Phyllis Goldberg and Rosemary Lichtman

Today more than 20 million Millennials aged 18-34 live with their parents. In tracking five different families as they navigate the generation gap between parents and boomerang kids, coaches Phyllis Goldberg and Rosemary Lichtman tap the creative power of story to give counsel and comfort. *Nonfiction*

Appendix

0 TO 5 MI TRAINING SCHEDULE					
week 1	week 2	week 3	week 4	week 5	week 6
walk daily, start with 1/2 mi, work up to 1 mi	walk daily, start with 1 mi, work up to 1 1/2 mi	walk daily, start with 1 1/2 mi, work up to 2 mi	work from 2 up to 3 mi at a stretch 5 days/wk	work from 3 up to 4 mi at a stretch 4 days/wk	work from 4 up to 5 mi at a stretch 4 days/wk
			2 days/wk mix your miles with intermittent walking activities	3 days/wk mix your miles with intermittent walking activities	3 days/wk mix your miles with intermittent walking activities

HIIT							
warm-up	fast walk/jog	sprint	fast walk/jog	sprint	fast walk/jog	sprint	cool down
5 min at 3.5 speed	2 min at 4.0 mi speed	1 min at 6.0 mi speed	2 min at 4.0 mi speed	1 min at 6.0 mi speed	2 min at 4.0 speed	1 min at 6.0 speed	4 min at 3.5 speed

5 TO 50 MILES TRAINING SCHEDULE						
	MON	TUE	WED	THURS	FRI	SAT	SUN
WEEK 1	Rest	Cross-training 45 min.	Walk-hike 3 miles	Weight training 30 min.	Cross-training 45 min.	Hike 5 miles	Walk-hike 3 miles
WEEK 2	Rest	Cross-training 45 min.	Walk-hike 3.5 miles	Weight training 30 min.	Cross-training 45 min.	Hike 6 miles	Walk-hike 3.5 miles
WEEK 3	Rest	Cross-training 1 hour	Hike 4 miles, 500 ft. elevation gain	Weight training 40 min.	Cross-training 1 hour	Hike 7 miles, 500 ft. elevation gain	Walk-hike 3 miles, 500 ft. elevation gain
WEEK 4	Rest	Cross-training 1 hour	Hike 4 miles, 500 ft elevation gain	Weight training 40 min.	Cross-training 1 hour	Hike 7 miles, 750 ft. elevation gain	Weight training 40 min.
WEEK 5	Rest	Cross-training 1 hour	Hike 4 miles, 500 ft. elevation gain	Weight training 40 min.	Cross-training 1 hour	Hike 8 miles, 1000 ft. elevation gain, carry 10 lbs.	Hike 3 miles, 500 ft. elevation gain, carry 10 lbs.
WEEK 6	Rest	Cross-training 1 hour	Hike 3 miles, 500 ft. elevation gain, carry 15 lbs.	Weight training 40 min.	Cross-training 1 hour	Hike 9 miles, 1250 ft. elevation gain, carry 15 lbs.	Hike 4 miles, 500ft. elevation gain, carry 15 lbs.

5 TO 50 MILES TRAINING SCHEDULE							
	MON	TUE	WED	THURS	FRI	SAT	SUN
WEEK 7	Rest	Weight training 1 hour	Hike 3 miles, 500 ft. elevation gain, carry 15 lbs.	Weight training 40 min.	Cross-training 1 hour	Hike 10 miles, 1500 ft. elevation gain, carry 20 lbs.	Hike 4 miles, 500 ft. elevation gain, carry 20 lbs.
WEEK 8	Rest	Cross-training 1 hour	Hike 3 miles, 500 ft. elevation gain, carry 20 lbs.	Weight training 40 min.	Cross-training 1 hour	Hike 12 miles, 2000 ft. elevation gain, carry 20 lbs.	Hike 4 miles, 500 ft. elevation gain, carry 20 lbs.

50 TO 500 MILES TRAINING SCHEDULE MONTH 3							
	MON	TUES	WED	THURS	FRI	SAT	SUN
WEEK 9	Rest from formal training	Weight training 40 min., stretch 15 min.	Hike 4 miles, 500 ft. elevation gain, carry 20 lbs. stretch	Weight training 40 min. stretch 15 min.	Cross-training, steady workout 1 hour	Hike 12 miles, 1500 ft. elevation gain, carry 25 lbs., stretch	Hike 5 miles, 500 ft. elevation gain, carry 15 lbs., stretch
WEEK 10	Rest	Weight training 40 min., stretch 15 min.	Hike 5 miles, 500 ft. elevation gain, carry 20 lbs.	Weight training 40 min. stretch 15 min.	Cross-training, steady workout 1 hour	Hike 12 miles, 2000 ft. elevation gain, carry 25-30 lbs. stretch	Hike 5 miles, 500-750 ft. elevation gain, carry 20 lbs. ,stretch
WEEK 11	Rest	Cross-training, steady workout 1 hour	Hike 4 miles, 500 ft. elevation gain, carry 15 lbs. stretch	Weight training 30 min. stretch 15 min.	Cross-training, steady workout 1 hour	Hike 10 miles, 1500 ft. elevation gain, carry 25-30 lbs.	Hike 4 miles, 500 ft. elevation gain, carry 20lbs. stretch
WEEK 12	Rest	Cross-training, easy steady workout 45 min.	Hike 3 miles, 500 ft. elevation gain, carry 20 lbs.	Weight training 20 min. stretch 15 min.	Cross-training, easy steady workout 45 min.	Hike 8 miles, 1000 ft. elevation gain, carry 20 lbs.	Hike 3 miles, 500 ft. elevation gain, carry 15 lbs.

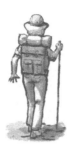

Backpacking Gear List

SLEEPING
- pillow
- tent + groundcloth, stakes
- sleeping pad
- sleeping bag
- waterproof stuff sack

CLOTHES:
- bras (2)
- buff
- down jacket
- 1 or 2 long sleeve shirts
- gloves (warm and fingerless ones)
- handkerchief (2)
- hat
- (zip off) hiking pants
- rain jacket
- short sleeve shirt
- long sleeve sun shirt
- sun hat
- socks (2)
- underwear (2)
- warm tights
- towel

EATING/KITCHEN
- bear canister, UR-sack
- bladder
- water bottle(s)
- cooking pot + cup
- food bag

- fuel
- pocket knife
- lighter
- spork
- stove
- (wind) screen
- pot scrubby + (soap)
- water purifying drops or tablets
- water filter

HYGIENE/MEDICAL
- alcohol wipes
- adhesive tape
- all purpose salve/lotion
- anti-inflammatory meds/aspirin
- band-aids/blister treatment
- (bug spray)
- comb/brush
- environmentally friendly soap
- floss (floss needles)
- (homeopathic remedies)
- hand sanitizer
- stretch bandage
- sterile gauze
- safety pins
- tweezers
- (scissors)
- sun screen
- toothpaste
- toothbrush
- toilet paper
- washrags (2)

Sources

Chapter 1

Silananda, S. U. "The Benefits of Walking Meditation."
Retrieved from http://www.accesstoinsight.org/lib/authors/
silananda/bl137.html

Chapter 3

Savage, L. E., Ph.D. "The Three Stages of a Woman's
Life." Retrieved from http://www.sandiegotherapists.com/
threestages.html

Gramann, S. 2015. "Menopause and Mood Disorders."
Retrieved from http://emedicine.medscape.com/
article/295382-overview.html

Lawrence-Lightfoot, S. 2009 *The Third Chapter: Passion,
Risk, and Adventure in the 25 Years After 50. Sarah Crichton
Books.*

Chapter 4

Dillard, A., The Writing Life. 2009. New York:
HarperCollins.

Levine, J., MD, PhD. Retrieved from https://www.getfit42.com/wp-content/uploads/2017/07/Stress_Management_And_Posture_Ebook_Final__UNSECURE_.pdf.

Infographic on Sitting Disease. Retrieved from http://www.juststand.org/tabid/674/language/en-US/default.aspx.

Bowman, K. 2014. Move Your DNA. Twin Lakes, WI: Lotus.

TED Talk on "Flow." Retrieved from https://www.ted.com/talks/mihaly_csikszentmihalyi_on_flow.

Csikszentmihalyi, M. 2008. Flow: The Psychology of Optimal Experience. New York: Harper Perennial.

Walser, R. 2013. The Walk. London: Serpent's Tail. http://walk2connect.com.

Chapter 5

Pittaway, K. Retrieved from http://besthealthus.com/wellness/healthy-habits/power-of-routines/.

Vernikos, J., PhD. 2011. Sitting Kills, Moving Heals. Fresno, CA: Quill Driver Books.

Chapter 7

Thoreau, H. D. 2010. Walking. Watchmaker Publishing, Ocean Shores WA

Capaldi C. A., R. L. Dopko, and J. M. Zelenski. 2014. "The Relationship Between Nature Connectedness and Happiness: A Meta-Analysis." Frontier Psychology 5: 976

Chapter 8

Haddock, D. 2001. Walking Across America in My Ninetieth Year. New York: Random House.

Lawrence Hunt, L. 2005. Bold Spirit. New York: Anchor Books.

Chapter 10

For more information on the Starlight 5Km program see http://www.legacyhealth.org/health-services-and-information/ wellness-and-prevention/couch-to-starlight-5k-training-program.aspx.

Reynolds, G. "A Way to Be Fit and Have Fun." Retrieved from http://well.blogs.nytimes.com/2015/07/29/a-way-to-get-fit-and-also-have-fun.

Brody, J. E. "Why Your Workout Should Be High Intensity." Retrieved from https://well.blogs.nytimes.com/2015/01/26/sweaty-answer-to-chronic-illness/?r=0&r=0.

Lunt, H., et al. "High Intensity Interval Training in a Real World Setting: A Randomized Controlled Feasibility Study in Overweight Inactive Adults, Measuring Change in Maximal Oxygen Uptake." Retrieved from http://www.ncbi.nlm.nih.gov/pubmed/24454698.

Karstoft, K., et al. "The Effects of Free-Living Interval-Walking Training on Glycemic Control, Body Composition, and Physical Fitness in Type 2 Diabetic Patients." Retrieved from http://www.researchgate.net/profile/SineKnudsen/publ ication/264850400TheEffectsofFree-LivingInterval-Walking TrainingonGlycemicControlBodyCompositionandPhysicalF itnessinType2DiabetesPatientsArandomizedcontrolledtrial/ links/53fb4d5a0cf20a4549706adf.pdf

Zuhl, M., and L. Kravitz. "HIIT vs. Continuous Endurance Training." Retrieved from https://www.unm.edu/lkravitz/ Article%20folder/HIITvsCardio.html.

Chapter 11
A walking shoe review: http://www.the-fitness-walking-guide.com/womens-walking-shoes.html.

Chapter 12
Schreiner, C. "Getting Some Miles in When Trails Aren't Nearby." Retrieved from http://blog.rei.com/hike/urban-hiking-getting-some-miles-in-when-trails-arent-nearby/.

Leicht, L. "Urban Hiking, the Most Epic Way to Burn Calories by Walking." Retrieved from http://dailyburn.com/life/fitness/urban-hiking-burn-calories-walking/.

Chapter 13
https://www.pacsafe.com/blog/10-best-urban-hiking-trails-in-america.html

For review of hiking shoes and boots, see Outdoor Gear Lab at http://www.outdoorgearlab.com/Hiking-Shoes-Womens-Reviews.

Chapter 16
"Sarcopenia with Aging." Retrieved from http://www.webmd.com/healthy-aging/sarcopenia-with-aging.

Loath, M. "Abnormal Gait." Retrieved from http://patient.info/doctor/abnormal-gait.

http://www.everydayhealth.com/fitness/how-fit-are-you-a-fitness-test-for-adults.aspx.

Vennare, J. "Test Your Strength: How Fit Are You Really?" Retrieved from http://dailyburn.com/life/fitness/best-fitness-tests-crossfit-marines/.

"10 Best Strength Training Exercises for Women Over

50." Retrieved from http://www.prevention.com/fitness/best-strength-training-exercises-women-over-50.

Reynolds, G. "3 Short Workouts or 1 Long One?" Retrieved from http://well.blogs.nytimes.com/2013/07/05/ask-well-3-short-workouts-or-1-long-one/.

Erickson, K. I., et al. 2011. "Exercise Training Increases Size of Hippocampus and Improves Memory." Proceedings of the National Academy of Sciences of the USA, Feb 108:7.

Andrews, C. G. "Take a Hike; Get a Bigger Brain." Retrieved from http://goodnature.nathab.com/take-a-hike-get-a-bigger-brain/.

Chapter 20

Simpson, K. M., B. J. Munro, and J. R. Steele. 2011. "Backpack Load Affects Lower Limb Muscle Activity Patterns of Female Hikers During Prolonged Load Carriage." Journal of Electromyography and Kinesiology 21 (5): 782–788.

"Fitting a Pack." Retrieved from http://www.rei.com/learn/expert-advice/backpacks-torso-hip-size.html.

For extensive gear lists with weight and product names, subscribe to Blackwoodspress.com.

Chapter 22

Michelson, M. "A Ghost Among Us." 2014. Backpacker (Aug): 95–104.

Chapter 23

Free PCT topo maps are available at https://www.pctmap.net/maps/.

Section 4

"Bear Incidents in the Sierras." Retrieved from http://www.
nps.gov/yose/planyourvisit/bearfacts.htm.

"SOS Signal." Retrieved from Wilderness Survival and
Safety website, http://www.chelansar.org.

Chapter 26

For more information on MBSR, see stress reduction.

Goyal, M., et al. 2014. "Meditation Programs for
Psychological Stress and Well-Being: A Systematic Review and
Meta-Analysis." JAMA Internal Medicine 174:357–368.

Brewer, J. "Mindfulness Training in the Military."
Retrieved from http://www.iflscience.com/brain/does-
mindfulness-physically-alter-cells-cancer-survivors0.

Zeidan, F., et al. 2012. "Mindfulness Meditation-Related
Pain Relief: Evidence for Unique Brain Mechanisms in the
Regulation of Pain." Elsevier Neuroscience Letters 520 (2):
165–173.

Donnelly, L. "A 25 minute walk could add 7 years to your
life." Retrieved from http://www.telegraph.co.uk/news/health/
news/11833720/25-minute-walk-could-add-7-years-to-life.
html.

Grant, J. A., et al. "Cortical Thickness and Pain Sensitivity
in Zen Meditators." Emotion 10:43–53.

Grant, J. A., et al. "A Non-Elaborative Mental Stance and
Decoupling of Executive and Pain-Related Cortices Predicts
Low Pain Sensitivity in Zen Meditators." Pain 152:150–156.

Strayed, C. 2013. Wild: From Lost to Found on the Pacific
Crest Trail. New York: Vintage Books.

Olson, S. "Brain Signals Behind Runner's High: Exercise-

Induced Euphoria Blocks Pain and Leads to Feeling Happy."
Retrieved from http://www.medicaldaily.com/brain-signals-
behind-runners-high-exercise-induced-euphoria-blocks-pain-
and-leads-350670.

Happy trails!

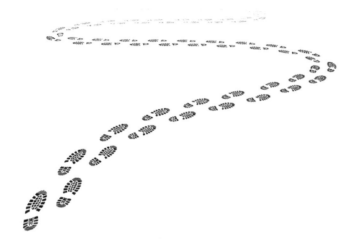

CPSIA information can be obtained
at www.ICGtesting.com
Printed in the USA
BVHW081516020519
547068BV00003B/263/P

9 780999 808924